Praise for Jim Bollenbach and *M*  *:
Stories from Inside the Musi*

"This book will open your eyes! Jim Bollenbacher, a formerly straight-laced attorney and corporate leader, shares his "retirement" as an event paramedic in jaw-dropping fashion. I laughed out loud in between gasps of astonishment at each story. Do yourself a favor, read about "this side" of the event/concert world. You'll laugh at, learn from and feel deeply grateful for Jim and his peers' experiences."

– Melanie Goldish, Author of *How Was Your Day, Baby?* and founder of SuperSibs

"Interesting tales of his experiences...covering the craziness of music festivals from the EMS perspective...funny stories that ring true...an enjoyable read about a little-known aspect of the EMS experience."

– Peter Canning, Author of *Paramedic: On the Front Lines of Medicine* and *Rescue 471: A Paramedic's Stories*

"Molly, Mushrooms, & Mayhem is a must-read for anyone considering a medical career. Author Jim Bollenbacher flawlessly compiled stories from fellow first responders that showcase the unpredictability of working in the field and display a remarkable sense of compassion for patients. Packed with hilarity, reflections of personal growth, off-the-wall encounters, and medical/EMS tidbits, this is one book that won't disappoint."

– Kerry Hamm, Author of The Real Stories from a Small-Town ER Series

"This is a great read that will give the average person some things to consider before going to their next festival, and the average EMT/Paramedic some things to consider before agreeing to work that next big event. If you have never done event/festival medicine you may find this book hard to believe. Having been there, done that, and cleaned the vomit-soaked shoes that prove it, it makes me smile and laugh because it's all true."

– Colleen Clark, Flight Nurse, CFRN, & Festival Nurse

MOLLY, MUSHROOMS, & MAYHEM

Stories from Inside the Music Festival
Medical Tent

Jim Bollenbacher

ISBN: 978-1-7352433-0-6

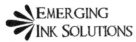 EMERGING
INK SOLUTIONS
Kara Scrivener, Editor
www.emergingink.com

Illustrations by Fionna Libby & Andreea Lulia Raicu
Images: 123rf.com/grebeshkovmaxim & bogdanhoda
Photography by Debbie Hassman, Treasuring Life's Moments
Photography

The stories within are true and accurate to the best of the author's
knowledge and the memories of the storytellers. Some creative
license has been taken to add color to settings or activities based on
in-field experience. The stories herein are offered without guarantee
on the part of the author, the storytellers, the editor/formatter, or the
book's press. The author disclaims all liability in connection with the
use of this book.

Notice: All medical teams described within the following work
followed applicable protocols and procedures as required at the time
of the incident. If it appears otherwise, it is due to the author's
writing, not the performance of the first responders. Names have
been changed and descriptions of settings and events have been
altered slightly to protect the privacy of patients.

This book is dedicated to every first responder who treats their patients with dignity and skill regardless of their ability to pay, the color of their skin, who they love, or what god they pray to.

INTRODUCTION

According to *Billboard* magazine, 32 million people attend music festivals every year. In 2017, more than 100,000 people attended each day of Coachella, bringing in over $100 million to the festival. The daily crowd at Lollapalooza in Chicago is larger than the population of all but five cities in Illinois. Since the inception of the music festival with Woodstock in 1969, such events have become big business. The appeal? A chance to see multiple bands over a long weekend and to party with family, friends, and like-minded strangers.

But there's another group of people who flock to the concerts – just not for the music. Known as "event paramedics," these people are medical professionals who tend to the many people at these large gatherings.

I know because I am one of them.

Unsurprisingly, the event-paramedic industry has also grown into big business. Entire companies now exist to provide medical care at overcrowded events. From bee stings and band-aids to overdoses and violence, the medical professionals play an important, but mostly hidden role.

I wrote this book because when I tell friends and family stories about my experiences as an event paramedic, they're either amazed, disgusted, or amused. Many times, they simply shake their heads in disbelief. These stories highlight what makes festivals both amazing and frightening. They also represent my passage from an inexperienced EMT to a seasoned and confident paramedic. Never would I have imagined myself in some of these situations back in the days when I was a lawyer. My wingtip shoes and Brooks Brothers suits would not have survived.

With the benefit of hindsight, I can share the humor and craziness from events that otherwise would have been grim. Of course, it's not my intention to downplay the possible risks involved in taking drugs or having a serious medical incident. In fact, I have worked at several large festivals where young adults have died. The impact of a death on the medical staff is palpable. I can't begin to imagine the effect on the families. Nevertheless, some unusual stuff happens within the medical tent that needs to be shared.

I want people to understand that these large events have dedicated medical professionals to care for anyone who needs help. Often, these professionals are volunteers and when they *are* paid, the wages are usually just above minimum wage. They are there because they love what they do and have a passion for service.

The stories contained herein come not only from me, but from EMTs and paramedics from around the country with many years of experience working at these kinds of events. The festivals remain unnamed out of respect for the event producers and the events themselves. I firmly believe that event producers go to great lengths to keep their events safe and the attendees healthy. If I thought otherwise, I would not continue to work for them, nor would many of my colleagues.

I hope as you read the following tales, you recognize and honor the role of first responders, many of whom are caring for victims of the COVID-19 pandemic today. They deserve our respect and support.

All profits from the sale of this book go to First Responders Children's Foundation supporting first responders and their families.

Enjoy.

IN THE BEGINNING

I was there to save the day, though from what, I did not yet know. My uniform was clean. My new blue EMT pants had nine pockets – yes, nine. To this day, I don't know what is supposed to go in them, but at the time, I was certain I looked the part of a Hollywood medic.

It was 2017 and I was working at my first music festival just weeks after obtaining my EMT license. It was also the first music festival I had *ever* attended. I was assigned to one of the main stages, which was run by a crusty old festival veteran who was in charge of the medical team, including me.

"Go stand over there," he told me in gruff voice.

I had no idea what I was about to experience, but I was excited to save my first patient.

A year earlier, I had retired from a professional career as a lawyer and business executive. I had been a suit-and-tie, sit-behind-a-desk-and-attend-meetings kind of guy. Physical labor, work boots, dirt, blood, and gore had never been part of my job description. In fact, I had taken an EMT class to simply fill my spare time. And I had fallen in love.

After getting my license, I was hired by a company that provides medical care at most of the major music festivals and many of the large sporting events in Chicago. That led me here, standing in the middle of a very large, grassy park surrounded by multiple stages featuring bands I had never heard of and tens of thousands of screaming fans about to descend on me. I was fired up.

Hours before the first band took the stage, the crowd came pouring in, running across the field to get a prime spot along the fence. Teens, 20-somethings, and older people were all desperate for the front row. For many, their primary objective was to see a band called The Killers, the headliner on my stage, which was scheduled to come on around 8:30 p.m.

It was 10:45 a.m. Suddenly, I felt very old.

To ensure crowd control and security, a fence was erected to block the crowd from the stage. That fencing ran along the front and into the crowd for about 50 yards, creating two separate L-shaped "pens" for the fans to fill. I was eventually assigned a position in the center aisle which divided them and gave VIPs access to prime viewing spots unmolested. It also gave me a pretty good view of the crowd. Two young EMT students were assigned to the same area; together we were determined to stop medical catastrophes before they arose.

It didn't take long before I saw a young woman in distress between music sets. She was at the back of the crowd on her knees. Hunched forward and very still, she had both hands on the sides of her head. Trouble. Her long blond hair prevented me from seeing her face, but it was obvious something was wrong. I called to her but got no response. I called again and still no response. Serious trouble. I climbed over a chest-high chain link fence with the grace of a 57-year-old.

Having picked up on my concern, the EMT students eagerly followed. I'm sure they thought they were going to learn something and have a cool story to tell in class. Approaching the woman, I ran through the systematic patient assessment in my head: airway, breathing, circulation. I recalled the questions I had been taught, though I was not entirely sure I had them right.

"Hi, my name is Jim. I'm an EMT," I said, kneeling. "Are you okay?"

My heart pounded as she turned to me.

"Yeah, I'm just talking to my mom, and this is the only way I can get a signal on my cell phone."

Well, look at me. Saving the world, one patient at a time.

It was an inauspicious start to my career in event medicine. Thankfully, my day improved and I was able to care for real patients. The entire experience was tiring, exhilarating, and eye-opening. I saw an unhappy patient spit at an EMT, people who had passed out, and others suffering from claustrophobia. I learned about The Killers, actually enjoyed some rap music, and saw a few celebrities in the flesh, relaxing and enjoying some down time.

More importantly, I fell in love with festival medicine – the rush of adrenaline, the call to the unknown, and the chaos of a large event. I was hooked. Of course, I had yet to be called to a patient in a porta-potty, but all in good time.

WHAT AM I DOING HERE?

I had always been curious about medical issues. I was the guy who slowed down passing a car accident, resisting the urge to jump out to help, and I loved watching reality medical shows on TV. My mom was a nurse, but I never had an interest in medicine when I was young. Science just wasn't my thing. I wanted to be an FBI agent until I met one who was a monumental jerk. So, I chose law school instead. What I liked most about being a lawyer was the adrenaline rush of being in the courtroom, not the tedium of law office work.

When I retired early, I came across an EMT class at our local community college and took it just for fun. My instructor was an amazing educator whom I'm certain I drove crazy with my incessant questions. He showed me the practical aspects of physiology and how the body works. His enthusiasm and knowledge unlocked something in me that made me excited about the possibility of a new career.

When the class ended and I got my EMT license, I took jobs in a local hospital emergency room and with a music and sports event medicine company. I enjoyed being an EMT and was able to see a lot in the ER, but my skills and knowledge were too limited to allow me to really do much. After a year, I decided that if I was going to pursue this, I needed the skills to work at a higher level. So, at age 60, I became one of the world's oldest paramedic students.

I went through the paramedic program at Northwest Community Hospital, which has the distinction of being the first paramedic program in Illinois. The head of the program is legendary for her knowledge and commitment to EMS teaching and our comprehensive course was 40 hours a week for the better part of 10 months. That included over 200 hours in the hospital and almost 700 hours on an ambulance. The absolute highlight of my training was getting to deliver a baby while working in Labor and Delivery. The doctor was right there with me, but the baby came into this world in my hands. It's hard to describe how amazing that felt. And seeing a cesarean section performed gave me newfound respect for both doctors and my wife.

I've discovered that the people in this profession are amazing. They are not just "ambulance drivers." They have life-saving skills and knowledge. I have also learned about the music festival culture, which was completely foreign to me.

Working at music festivals keeps me young. It's down and dirty, and it's an adrenaline rush. Every call can provide the tension and challenge of a Supreme Court argument, even if I eventually find out that the "emergency" is a naked man in the wrong camp. I love the chaos, the challenge, and the people. I love that I get dirty and sweaty instead of sitting behind a desk in an office. And I love that this work calls for the same kind of analysis and problem solving that being a lawyer or business leader required, only faster. People's lives are literally in your hands.

I was at the point in my life where I was ready to give back, to do something I felt really good about without worrying about the paycheck. I've been blessed to work with some really special people, but my EMT and paramedic colleagues are unparalleled. Their skill and dedication at these festivals, and elsewhere, is remarkable, and I am in awe of them.

There's one small issue though: I don't really care for the music at most of these events. My musical tastes are stuck in the seventies and eighties. My daughters listened to music and went to concerts, but I don't recall what or who they liked or whether that included EDM (Electronic Dance Music). Thankfully, I didn't know then what I know now about music festivals or I wouldn't have allowed them to attend. That was the old conservative me though.

When I first started out, I needed some musical help and my daughters tried their best.

"What's EDM?" I asked.

"It's like a DJ, Dad, but they make their own music. And it's electronic, not instruments."

"Don't DJs play records of other people's music?" I asked.

"Records, Dad? Really?"

That was then. I have since learned quite a bit about EDM by working at the festivals. First, it's not my thing. Second, it's really loud. And third, the artists are incredibly talented. I recently described EDM to a friend this way: "It's like the old-fashioned DJs, but they make their own music, it's all electronic, and they have amazing light shows. And it makes my head hurt." That's growth, right?

To be at one of these festivals is an experience unlike much else. Tens of thousands of people come together to enjoy music, dance with arms raised, and celebrate life. Like rock was in the seventies, EDM is more than a type of music; it's a culture with a modern hippie aesthetic of glitter, headbands, and beads that celebrates diversity. Its mantra is Peace, Love, Unity, and Respect or PLUR.

To me, it's like Woodstock with cell phones. Attendees roam from stage to stage picking their favorites from the menu of shows. The first time I saw people crowd-surfing a young woman across the top of the crowd, I was both mortified and jealous. I shuddered at the thought of my daughters doing it. Yet I realized these kids were having fun in a way I could never have imagined in my youth.

For the medical staff, music festivals present unique challenges. Regardless of the weather, we're outside with large crowds of people often in remote locations. Festival attendees are generally younger and perhaps more prone to errors of judgment in their exuberance than they might otherwise be. Our equipment is limited and our "hospital" is a tent with cots. We don't deal with our patients in the back of an ambulance or in an ER. Festival medicine is unique and the people I work with love it. I've met great young adults just trying to have fun with their friends. And many, many of them make a point of thanking us for being there. I almost always come away from a festival feeling both exhausted and refreshed.

That is the *new* me. The old me grew up in a conservative, blue-collar home in western Pennsylvania where drugs and alcohol were definitely not an acceptable choice.

My views on drug use were also heavily influenced by the hippie era. Only *those people* used drugs and were seen as ne'er-do-wells. It had also been a time when rumors of Vietnam veterans returning from war addicted to drugs like heroin flourished. No thanks, I thought.

These days, I don't advocate the use of illegal drugs, but neither do I condemn the way these young adults choose to live and have fun.

YOLO (You Only Live Once), right?

And of the millions of them showing up to dance, and hug, and share their love of music, only a very small percentage need our help. They are the stars of this book.

Becoming an Emergency Medical Technician, or EMT, is the first level of training for medical emergencies. EMTs receive about 120-150 hours of classroom and clinical training while paramedics have more advanced training which generally includes at least 1,200-2,000 hours in class, skills lab, hospital clinicals, and ambulance training.

In most states, paramedics are able to perform advanced lifesaving procedures such as intubation, correct cardiac arrythmias, and administer numerous medications.

WHO IS THIS MOLLY PERSON?

"All right, brain. You don't like me, and I don't like you, so let's just do this and I'll get back to killing you with beer." – Homer Simpson

I admit that I smoked marijuana as a young adult, particularly in law school. What can I say? School was stressful and that was the popular drug of choice when we wanted to relax and have a good time. But the recreational drug use stopped once I entered the workforce. I never did "hard" drugs and didn't know anyone who did, so when I began working as paramedic, MDMA ("Molly"), acid, ketamine ("Special K"), combined ecstasy or LSD, and mushrooms ("hippy flipping") were all foreign to me.

I vividly recall my first night at a large EDM festival, where my partner and I talked at length to some attendees about the drugs and all the terminology. I was stunned by how little I knew. I can't say I was appalled because I didn't know what I didn't know. Mostly I didn't understand why drug use was a thing at these festivals. Why not just have a beer and enjoy the music? I had a lot to learn.

In my opinion, festival owners go to great lengths to provide a safe environment, even having security perform pat downs and using drug-sniffing dogs at the entrance gates. But people are very creative about ways to smuggle drugs into an event. I watched a young man come through security at the entrance innocently wearing a D.A.R.E. T-shirt. After he was cleared through security, he ran to a group of his friends and pulled a big bag of weed from deep inside the crotch of his pants. Well played, young man, well played.

In a small number of cases, that creativity can lead to a trip to the medical tent. Most of the time, the person just needs to be hydrated or to sleep and recover. Other times, drug use causes a serious medical issue. It leads to some very funny, crazy, or gross stories that the patients probably wish to forget. But we remember.

My Initiation

"Better on the brain than on the plane." That's the mindset I was told to expect. It was the last show on the final night of my first EDM festival, and if you had any drugs or alcohol left, that was the time to use them up. The performing artist was known to put on an amazing show with incredible light and video displays. His shows were also known for resulting in a significant number of medical emergencies. Was it the lights, the timing, the size of the crowd? All I knew was that we were going to be busy and so had positioned a number of teams around the venue to be ready for the inevitable.

Shortly after the performance started, my team received a call about a hostile patient at the back of the crowd. When we got there, a young woman ran up to us and said that her friend in the crowd was having a seizure. My partner was an experienced paramedic so he told me he would take the hostile patient since he could sedate him if necessary. I should go find the person having seizures. I followed the woman deep into the crowd until we found her friend lying on her side with another woman kneeling beside her.

"Hi, what happened?" I yelled over the thumping bass

"She was just sitting there watching the show and I looked over and she was having a seizure," one of the women told me.

"Okay, are you sure it was a seizure?" I asked.

"Yeah, I'm sure. I'm a nurse. She definitely had a seizure."

"Great, thanks. Do you know if she took anything?"

"I think some Molly," she said.

"Are you sober?"

"No."

When someone faints, people often describe what happened as a seizure, so it was helpful that she had the medical background to recognize a seizure. It was also important that she not be seen caring for the patient after she had been drinking or using drugs, so I told her that she should leave as soon as help arrived to avoid any problems. She had been helpful to me and I didn't want her to get in any kind of trouble.

As we finished this conversation, the patient started seizing again. She was already on her side, so there was not much more to do other than make sure she did not hurt herself. Because my partner had our bags, the only equipment I had with me was a flashlight. I contacted dispatch.

"Dispatch, this is Team Two. I'm with a patient who is seizing."

"Team Two, repeat."

It was extremely loud and I had a hard time hearing dispatch in my earpiece just as they had trouble hearing me. "I am in the crowd with a patient actively seizing," I shouted.

"Where are you, Team Two?"

I tried to describe my location, but we were far enough into the crowd and down a hill that I could not see much more than people dancing. I tried to pinpoint my location in the huge crowd, but the truth was I had no idea. After a few unsuccessful tries to get help, dispatch informed me that they didn't have any available units and that I needed to do the best I could until someone freed up.

Well, dandy.

Here I was in the middle of a raucous crowd with a nurse who was high and all the medical teams were tied up. As a lawyer, I was confident in my ability to help solve my client's problems. At that moment though, as a new EMT alone with my patient, I had little faith in my ability to care for this young woman. Fortunately, her seizure lasted only about 30 seconds at which point she slowly started to become coherent. But I still had to get her out of the crowd and somewhere help could find us.

She was very petite, so I picked her up in my arms, asked someone to clear the way for me, and began carrying her up the hill out of the crowd. It was a great idea, except the hill was a lot steeper on the way up than it had seemed on the way down. And I was not exactly in tiptop shape.

Halfway up, I regretted my decision and began praying I didn't drop this poor lady. When I finally reached the top of the hill, I saw a woman sitting on a queen-sized air mattress.

I yelled to her, "Hey, *(gasp!)* I'm medical *(gasp!)*. I need your mattress."

I did not wait for a response and placed the young woman on the mattress. Its owner was either happy to help or too intoxicated to care. My patient was more alert now and doing well. I, on the other hand, needed oxygen.

I learned later that calls for medical assistance were coming in about every 60 seconds. That explained why I had ended up on my own. Eventually, help arrived and we got the patient to the medical tent where she made a full recovery.

What an initiation.

As I've looked back on that call, I've realized that, despite my doubts, I did what I needed to do and my patient was fine. Perhaps it was divine providence or luck, but I attribute it to great training.

That training, and my confidence, continue to be tested with each new call.

———

When you see someone having a seizure, turn them on their side so they don't choke or inhale secretions into their lungs. Never put anything into a person's mouth while they are seizing. Being in the field and getting real calls is very different from practicing scenarios in a classroom. And that is scary as hell.

———

Molly Mayhem
As Told by Lindsay (Paramedic)

Lil Pump, LL Cool J, and Gucci Mane performed back-to-back on two stages that were catty-corner from each other. Who could possibly have thought that was a good idea? We knew it was going to be bad. But even we had no idea.

I was part of a field team, assigned to wander through the crowd and assist anyone in need. I had no idea who the hell Lil Pump was. I figured he was some C-List rapper who had been booked to fill space. But as the day went on, more and more people explained to me that this guy was the reason they had come to the festival. *Okay*, I thought, *if you say so.*

For most of the day, the crowds were fairly well-behaved. It was hot, so I expected more patients with heat exhaustion or who were stupid drunk. We were deployed backstage and as we waited for a call, I could see a rapidly growing mass in front of the stage. The crowd was becoming louder and rowdier with each passing minute.

The second the artist skipped onto the stage, the crowd lost its minds. A pulsating mass of teenagers surged forward and bounced to the bass, encouraged by the rapper and his crew. With that surge, problems escalated. Unconscious concert-goers were pulled up and over the barriers. The ones who could walk were assisted off to the side while the others were carried or pushed on a stair chair. All I could do was stand there, slack-jawed, and watch as security struggled to get the frenzy under control. By now, the crowd had doubled in size.

Suddenly, security grabbed me, yelling for a medic.

A burly man guided us to a kid lying on the ground. He was shirtless, hot to the touch, pale, and drenched in sweat. Without asking, I knew he had taken Molly; his eyes were dilated to the size of dinner plates.

"Hey man, what's going on? You okay?" I asked.

His eyes were glazed and he looked through me rather than at me. "I'm *awesome!*" he yelled.

I rolled my eyes. Of course, he was.

"Yeah dude, you don't look awesome. What'd you take?"

"Nothing," he replied.

It's always nothing.

"I'm not the cops. I just need to know what you took so I can help you."

"I'm on Moh-hol-ly!" he screamed in a sing-song voice with a crazed smile on his face.

"I bet you are," I laughed. "How old are you, my man?"

"I'm 16," he replied, throwing up his fingers in the rock n' roll horns.

Shit. Underage. Immediate transport needed.

"Maaaaaan, you should be at home applying for college or doing homework, not out here doing Molly!"

I had my partner radio in for transport, but we were met with an overworked dispatcher. "Yeah, you and everyone else at that stage. Just sit tight," dispatch replied.

I could tell the kid was overheating. Taking Molly on a hot August day while being crushed between 5,000 of your closest friends was asking for a heat stroke or seizure. Not what I wanted in the middle of a rap concert. I grabbed a bottle of water and started pouring it over him. He writhed and moaned in ecstasy.

"Oh my *God*, that feels sooo *goooood*! Yeeesssss!" he screamed.

I paused, weirded out by his reaction, but shrugged and continued to pour water down his chest and abdomen. He continued to moan and make weird sex noises as I did my best to cool him down. Eventually, my partner and I carried him out of the mud and onto the stair chair, moving him off to the side to wait for transport.

I kept trying to push a bottle of water into his hand and encourage him to drink, but every couple of minutes, he lost focus and started spilling it everywhere, causing him to again moan like he was having an orgasm. The music cut out behind me. The crowd groaned and protested loudly. Apparently, the rapper's equipment had overheated; the show was over.

We eventually got the transport cart we needed and the kid was taken to the main medical tent. My colleagues were all in a daze, shell-shocked, and exhausted. We probably looked like zombie soldiers returning from a particularly bloody apocalypse.

Molly, also known as ecstasy or "E," is a drug called MDMA which stands for methylenedioxymethamphetamine — in other words, it has methamphetamine in it. It increases the amount of the feel-good hormone serotonin in the brain, which causes the sensation of emotional closeness and empathy. It is also a stimulant and can cause increased physical activity, which can lead to a dangerous rise in core body temperature. It may also lower the body's seizure threshold.

Hi Daddy

Sometimes medical emergencies don't find us; we find them. I was driving a golf cart at an event when my colleagues and I saw a large crowd of people gathered at a crossing manned by security. We flipped on our siren for a second to get people's attention so they could clear the way. Instead, security came up to us and told us they had a very confused woman who needed attention. The crowd included her friends and concerned strangers.

The woman was clearly disoriented and having trouble getting from point A to point B. For her safety, she needed to be in the medical tent, where she could be seen by a doctor. We placed her securely on the backboard of the cart with her head to the back. She was very compliant, even talkative, and gave us no trouble. I sat in the rear-facing seat and was able to monitor her.

"Hi, Daddy," she said.

Huh?

She was looking right at me. "I'm sorry, Daddy."

"No, I'm not your daddy. I'm an EMT," I said.

"Okay, Daddy."

"Hey, what's your name?" I asked. "Do you know where you are?"

"Yes, Daddy. I'm having fuuunnnn!!"

At first, I thought she was joking with me because I was easily old enough to be her father. But it became obvious as this continued that she believed I was her father. She was both happy to see me and concerned I would be angry with her. I didn't play along with her hallucination – that's not a good idea – but assured her that I wasn't upset and was only interested in making sure she was okay.

When we arrived outside the medical area, she quite vocally told my colleagues that I was her dad and asked to put her arm around me as we walked into the tent. It was quite a scene and I received a fair amount of abuse from them later. Inside the tent, one of our security guards helped her onto the cot so she could be checked out and then sleep off whatever she had taken.

I was kneeling beside her when she reached into her bra and pulled out a crumpled roll of what seemed to be a lot of cash. The security guard misunderstood her intentions.

"No hon, we don't need your money. This is all free," the security guard assured her.

She smiled, looked at me, and said, "Give it to my dad so he can keep it safe."

I laughed out loud, but the security guard was confused. She then reached back into her bra and pulled out a clear plastic baggie with an assortment of pills in it.

"Here, Daddy," she said, "I don't need these anymore."

She then turned on her side and went to sleep. We kept her cash safe and returned it to her when she sobered up. Her bag of pills went into the "amnesty box" where we kept drugs given to us by patients until we could dispose of them. I have often wondered how that young woman felt the next day when she realized that she had two more days at the music festival but had given away her bag of drugs.

Getting Lit
As Told by Josh (Paramedic)

My partner and I were on our way to a call, driving our cart on paths that led from the spectators' area into off-limits grounds. As medical staff, we had wristbands that gave us access to almost every part of a festival and we used those off-limits areas to get to patients more quickly than if we had to go through a crowd. It was the first time I had worked this festival, and also my very first call. I was an inexperienced EMT, so this was new to me.

As we drove, we came across a young woman who was rolling in the dirt in the middle of the path. She was also topless. I don't recall if her wristband allowed her to be there, but given her behavior, I suspected she was not.

We stopped to see what was going on and heard her saying to no one in particular, "It's gonna be lit. It's gonna be lit." When we asked her questions, her response each time was the same.

"Hi, what's your name?" I asked.

"I don't know. Let's find out," she replied in a sing-song cadence.

"What are you doing?"

"I don't know. Let's find out."

"Did you take anything today?"

"I don't know. Let's find out."

We radioed dispatch and asked them to send another team to our original call. This woman needed some medical care. We sat her up and tried to cover her with a tarp to keep her out of public view as much as possible. When we examined her, she did not appear to have any injuries and her vital signs were all normal. But she was convinced that something was "gonna get lit."

We put her in the rear-facing seat of the cart and buckled her in; I rode next to her. I did my best to keep her covered by the tarp, but she kept pushing it off as she boosted herself in the seat.

"It's gonna be lit."

We made it to medical with her still in her seat and mostly covered. We dropped her off in the care of the doctors and nurses there and that was the last I heard of her. I'm sure she recovered when the drugs wore off and had a great time the rest of the weekend.

I never did "find out" what was "gonna be lit."

—————

I have often thought that being an older paramedic has both benefits and challenges. Most of the people I deal with assume I've been doing this for a while and that I know what I am doing. That's not always the case. However, being older than most patients does allow me to be more persuasive than if I were a baby-faced 22-year-old. And my life experience allows me to understand situations with a different perspective than I would have when I was younger.

In my years as an adult and father, I have seen and experienced many of the things my patients are going through, which allows me to feel a level of empathy I otherwise would not have felt. On the downside, it's a physical job and years behind a desk have made me soft. Fortunately, most of my younger colleagues take pity on me and help me out – usually right after a snide comment on my age. Even so, the calls in the next few stories challenged me physically and made me feel my age.

Mushroom Mania

Before I worked at music festivals, I had heard of – but never experienced – the impact of mushrooms firsthand. Not the kind you find in a salad or on a steak, but the psychedelic type. I wasn't even sure that "mushrooms" were really mushrooms or just a slang term to describe a drug.

In fact, these are *real* mushrooms that can be found in the wild or cultivated and contain a substance called psilocybin, a well-known hallucinogen. They can be dried, eaten, smoked, or used to make tea that sends you on a hallucinogenic "trip." I still haven't seen an actual 'shroom, but I've seen what they can do. It's one of the drugs that worries me the most.

My mushroom education began at one of the smaller EDM festivals which took place in a city park and had about 25,000 in attendance each day. Four stages dotted the park, which was fenced off to prevent non-festival-goers from entering. In addition to "field teams," teams of two people with medical bags, we also had two teams on designated four-wheel carts to transport patients. I was on one of those four-wheelers when my partner and I were called to a stage; security had a patient for us.

This was not an uncommon type of call, and usually meant we would find someone who was being aggressive and 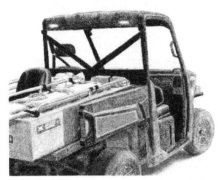 out of control. In this case, we arrived to find a young man sitting cross-legged on the ground. Security observed him on his hands and knees just outside the large crowd, crawling along the earth, picking imaginary items off the ground and out of the air. When they checked on him, he hadn't responded, so they were concerned for his well-being. When we met him, he was continuing to pick up invisible items from the grass.

He was docile and completely happy to ride with us on our cart to the medical tent. Sitting between my partner and I on the front bench seat, he seemed content in his own space. Unfortunately for us, at several points along the way, he saw items in our path that caused him to scream and attempt to jump from the cart, fearing we were going to crash into them. Of course, there were no such items in our path. We held him between us, assuring him that he was safe as long as he stayed in the cart.

When we arrived at the medical tent, we laid him on a cot so we could assess his vital signs and complete some intake paperwork. We heard him talking to someone, presumably about the day's events. The conversation lasted for close to 10 minutes before a doctor came over to see what was going on.

The doctor's concern? There was no one with the patient, apart from his hallucination. He carried on a remarkable two-way conversation during which he both asked and answered a number of questions. Had someone been sitting next to him, it would have all seemed totally normal. But he was totally alone.

My next experience with mushrooms was at a larger festival, where approximately 40,000 people camped overnight. The campgrounds were large and spread out, mostly in open grassy fields, some in more wooded areas. Because of the camping, we had medical coverage on-duty 24-hours-a-day once the campers arrived. And on the night shift, when the shows were over, the excitement moved to those campgrounds. Informal parties blossomed everywhere while buses with DJs stationed atop their rooves played music for the crowds so people could continue to dance to the thumping beat.

Sometime after midnight, we were called to one of the campgrounds for an unknown issue. My partner and I drove to the location of the call in a golf cart and found ourselves in a small clearing in a wooded area. It was remote and not heavily trafficked by festival goers, at least not at that time. When we arrived, we were met by a "security" guard who was really there more to give directions and look for any problems. We also saw our patient: a large, very muscular man who was hugging his very petite wife.

"Hey, what's going on?" I asked.

"It's my husband. He did four grams of mushrooms," she replied.

I turned to my partner. "Is that a lot?"

He didn't know. I later learned it was.

I asked the woman if she had taken any.

"Yeah, but not as much," she said. "I'm okay, but I'm worried about him. This doesn't usually happen."

I could see that he had his eyes closed and seemed frozen in place. He did not acknowledge, respond to, or even appear to know we were there. They were locked in a lover's embrace; the rest of the world didn't seem to exist to him. Unfortunately, as we spoke to him, he grew more tense. I could see his facial expressions change to a mixture of fear and anger. Given how remote we were - and how big and strong he appeared to be, not to mention disassociated from reality - I was concerned for our safety.

One of the basic tenets of being an EMT or paramedic is to ensure our safety first. That is always the priority, not for selfish reasons, but practical ones. If we go into a dangerous scene and are injured, not only have we reduced the number of people who can help, we have added ourselves to the mix. In every practice scenario, we always began with "Is the scene safe?" Coming from an office job, it took me a while to fully appreciate the potential dangers I faced, but my appreciation of "scene safe" has grown.

In fact, violence against paramedics and EMTs is an increasing problem. The U.S. Centers for Disease Control and Prevention estimates that more than 2,000 EMTs and paramedics are injured every year. At music events, people are generally in good moods and recognize the value we bring to the scene; in addition, there is usually very good security. Other than my muscular friend on mushrooms, I don't recall being in a situation where I feared for my safety. But I'm always mindful of it and have become proficient at talk-down techniques. Convincing a patient to do something they don't want to do but need to do takes a balance of patience and compassion. Both are skills I rarely used as a lawyer. But as I've learned, a safe scene can take an unexpected turn when drugs or alcohol are involved and talking only goes so far.

In this case, I asked the security guard to call for more help but request that they come quietly. The last thing I wanted to do was panic our patient.

As we talked with his wife and attempted to talk to him, his embrace became tighter and tighter until he was squeezing her uncomfortably hard. I could see the worry on her face as he failed to respond to her pleas and our requests to let her go. I became concerned for her safety. She couldn't escape his iron embrace; it was increasingly difficult for her to breathe. The time for trying to talk him down had passed.

I drew up a syringe of ketamine based on my estimate of his weight, and somehow, while I was doing that, my partner and security got the couple on the ground where I was able to inject him. Ketamine works fast and it was but a few moments before he relaxed and released his grip on his wife. All of us breathed a sigh of relief. I immediately started an IV in his hand and flushed through an additional small dose. As fast as ketamine takes effect, it wears off, and I could not afford to have this giant of a man wake up as we transported him to medical. I also wanted to run some fluid into him to get him hydrated.

Several hours later, I met the couple again in the medical tent. He was awake, alert, and a very nice, gentle man. His wife was sitting on his lap and both were grateful for our help. He apologized for causing us trouble and after being fully evaluated by the doctors, went back to his camp for some early morning sleep. Between the remnants of the mushrooms and the ketamine, I suspect he had some pretty interesting dreams.

Ketamine was one of the first drugs I saw at music festivals. It can be used in small doses to control pain and in larger doses for sedation. Its properties make it a generally safe drug to use on an unruly or over-excited person. Unfortunately, it is also used recreationally (snorted like cocaine) to enhance the music festival experience because it produces a type of out-of-body sensation.

Anger Management
As Told by Josh (Paramedic)

We were called out to respond to reports of a woman behaving unusually. These kinds of calls are pretty common and most often result in us simply bringing the person to the medical tent to be assessed and monitored. This woman was in someone else's camp and wouldn't leave. No one knew who she was or what she was doing.

Initially, the woman appropriately answered all of our questions but she really didn't want anything to do with us. Then she grabbed at us, attempting to grope and kiss me and my partner. We moved her away and tried to redirect her focus so we could convince her to come with us to have a doctor look at her. She didn't like that idea and took off running, saying something about her campsite.

For our safety, we did not give chase but stayed on scene, letting dispatch know what was going on. We saw her run to the next camp and sit down in a chair directly in front of an RV. A guy showed up claiming to know her and walked over to the RV. We took this as good news, thinking we might get some information that could help us, or he could walk her back to her campsite to sleep it off. Instead, he began to kiss her neck and rub up and down her body. Given how out of it she appeared, this display made me very uncomfortable. My partner and I walked over and asked the young man to back away from her.

At this point, she was barely responsive and on the verge of passing out. As we questioned lover-boy, we smelled the pungent odor of booze waft from him; he was unable to answer any questions about the woman, including her name. He continued to try to caress her, so I pulled him away and called for supervisors and security.

Just then, an SUV pulled up. The people inside all seemed to know the guy trying to fondle my patient. As he and his friends in the SUV talked, my partner and I went to the woman and tried to pick her up to move her to our cart. We got her to her feet and, as I was supporting her with my shoulder under her arm, she balled up her fist and punched me in the face.

Where the hell did that come from?

I let go of her, pushing her away as she tried to kick me. My partner tackled her to the ground as I went to my bag and drew up a dose of ketamine. I was pissed and not going to mess around anymore. She was hostile enough to hurt us or herself. So, I gave her a shot in her thigh. Within 30 seconds, she was out "in the K-hole," as they say.

That is usually the end of these stories because once patients are non-violent, we put them on our backboard and off we go to medical. In this case though, as we drove, I noticed that she had developed trismus, or lockjaw. Her mouth was shut tight and nothing was going to open it. I had never seen this as a side effect of ketamine and I had no idea what other drugs she had taken. This was worrisome because if she happened to stop breathing, it was going to be difficult to open an airway to help her breathe. I told my partner to step on it; I hovered over her for the rest of the trip making sure she was okay.

Fortunately, she kept breathing and I did too. She spent some nap time in the medical tent and then left happy and healthy to enjoy the rest of the festival.

That's Trippy
As Told by Nathan (EMT)

I was working on the ambulance at an indoor EDM concert during the winter when one of our EMT teams brought a young woman to the medical area. She appeared to have taken ketamine and had been found lying on the floor of the event, staring at the ceiling, saying, "Purple, purple, purple, yellow, yellow, yellow..." over and over as the stage lights changed.

The concert was held in a large ballroom but was crowded with dancers and partiers. When they realized what the woman was doing, they began to prompt her with other things to say, most of which were stupid, funny, or dirty. When she found a phrase she liked, she would grab onto it and repeat it over and over. We learned accidentally that when someone said the word "trippy," she would yell out, "*Trippy!*" and throw her legs up in the air over her head and laugh. Even I had to admit we found it funny.

We put her on our ambulance stretcher, but had to restrain her with soft restraints for her safety. She was not combative, but in her altered state, she would not stay on the stretcher. Trying to get up and walk around in a moving ambulance wasn't safe for her, or us. Once in the ER, we suggested to the nurse that they keep her restrained, but the charge nurse told us it would be fine. So, we unlashed the woman.

The patient remained well-behaved as we gave the nurse our handover report describing the patient's condition. That report included her vital signs, the interventions we had performed, and a description of what had occurred at the concert.

"She was repeating words over and over and was disoriented," I explained. "And she really likes the word *trippy* for some reason."

As if on cue, the patient yelled "*Trippy,*" swung her legs in the air, and kicked the charge nurse in the face.

On went the hospital restraints.

She's Hot
As Told by Jon (EMT)

At outdoor festivals, medical teams are dispersed according to the layout of the venue. At this festival, which covered a very large space, we had EMTs and paramedics posted at each stage. In most cases, and in this case, there is a space between the fence containing the crowd and the stage where security, media, photographers, and medical are located.

I was positioned at the front of the crowd stage-left when I noticed a woman who appeared to be in her late-thirties fighting with another audience member. She was in the front and near a gate that allowed authorized people to move in and out of the crowd. Security was there trying to break up the fight, but the woman just started fighting them.

I grabbed my partner and went over to help. She was big enough, and wild enough, that it took four of us to control her. We ended up each taking a limb and, as she continued to thrash around, carried her up a small hill to an auxiliary medical tent manned by an experienced paramedic.

Patients brought to this medical tent are usually put onto a cot and treated for minor issues. If there is something serious, they are moved to the primary tent where they can be evaluated and treated by doctors and nurses. There was no way this patient was going to stay on a cot, so we laid her on the ground and tried to get her under control as she continued to writhe around and scream at us.

During the struggle, I noticed that her skin was extremely hot to the touch, much more so than the level of activity merited. This can be an ominous sign that someone's core temperature is dangerously high and a sign of a possible overdose of Molly. We needed to calm her and get her cooled down, or she ran the risk of seizures.

At this point, we had pretty much her entire body covered trying to control her. She was still fighting, kicking, and struggling. I was amazed at her strength and stamina but worried about her temperature. I yelled to the medic in the tent, "Dave, we need some Versed. She's burning up." The medic quickly drew up five milligrams of Versed and gave her an injection in the thigh. She calmed down enough that we were able to get the ambulance crew and their stretcher to us and load her on it.

My advice was to get her to the ER quickly, which they did. One of the EMTs from another team who had shown up halfway through this craziness, looked at me and asked, "What the hell was that all about?" All I could do was shake my head and walk back down the hill to await my next call.

All in a day's work at a music festival.

"That's Trippy" is a good example of how my views have evolved; I've become much more understanding of this culture. The young woman was clearly altered from drug use, and in the past, I would have frowned on her behavior. But she was happy and enjoying life at that moment in a way I'm not sure I ever have. I have never stared at the colors of the lights and had as much fun as she was having. She wasn't angry or hostile; she wasn't creating drama or trauma. She was quite happy to be with her caretakers. That is a common theme with many of our patients.

So, are my old-fashioned views about these things valid?

Should I re-evaluate how I feel about these things and be a little less judgmental?

IS IT ALWAYS THIS CRAZY?

"I may be crazy, but it keeps me from going insane." – Waylon Jennings

Look online for any music festival video and you'll see people doing things you don't normally see in your everyday life: dancing, sitting on friends' shoulders, wearing – or not – funky festival clothes, and sleeping under a tree in the middle of a field. Those are the more typical sights. What you might not see are the unusual incidents that get *our* attention. Funny, outlandish, embarrassing, and just plain weird are all in our sweet spot. The sense of freedom from 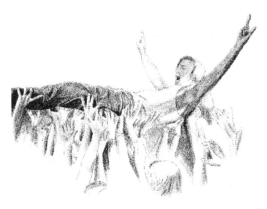 being outdoors away from work, parents, and loved ones can inspire all manner of out-of-the-norm behaviors. Throw in some alcohol, a few party drugs, and a sense of anonymity, and you get the stories in this book.

When I started this work, the consequences of the craziness bothered me. Festivals seemed irresponsible and excessive, putting a lot of people at risk. Even as a teenager, I didn't behave that way. The first time I went into a porta-potty for a patient was awful. It was hard to be understanding of the underage teen who had had too much to drink and threw up on me. But with each festival, I have learned to balance those few incidents with the majority of people who are having fun, behaving appropriately (or close to it), and are safe.

I made mistakes myself when I was young. Some were spectacular. You likely did as well. I remind myself that I signed up to take care of sick people. Therefore, I've learned some tricks of the trade. For instance, never stand directly in front of a sick patient. It puts you in the line of fire – I learned that one the hard way. Always have a vomit bucket and hand sanitizer with you and learn to recognize that moment when the vomit is about to fly. It's all good. I've adjusted and maybe, just maybe, I'm getting soft in my old age. Except for the porta-potties.

So Jim, what kind of crazy things *have* you and your colleagues encountered at these wild music festivals?

I'm so glad you asked.

Cheating Death
As Told by Nathan (EMT) and Pam (Paramedic)

"I don't feel well," declared a young man entering the medical tent where I was stationed. He was with his girlfriend, a young petite blonde who seemed worried.

It's not unusual for someone to bring themselves to the medical tent because it's always very visible and attendees know they can come in and be examined. We often have people bring their friends to us out of concern for them.

This young man appeared to be sober, or at least mostly so, and wasn't bleeding or vomiting, so I directed him to a cot and let the nurse know he was there. A few minutes later, the nurse yelled to me, "We need to get this guy on the monitor! His heart rate's almost 200."

Well, that explains why he didn't feel well.

When your heart is beating that fast, you can become lightheaded, among other things. In time, your heart will wear out and stop. This was a pretty significant issue for us, and him.

Our first response when we have a patient like that is to have them do a vagal maneuver, which consists of bearing down very hard for 15 seconds as if you are having a bowel movement. That movement can stimulate the vagal nerve and slow the heart rate.

29

When it works. It doesn't have a high rate of success, which means the patient either needs medication, or in the worst case, an electrical shock to reset the heart.

We explained all of this to the young man, whose only response was, "I can't go to the hospital."

"Okay, but this is really serious. You can't keep this up forever."

He seemed to understand but repeated that he couldn't go to the hospital. He desperately wanted us to help him "do that vagal thing." Fine, let's do it. He tried several times, straining to slow his heart rate with no success. We had him blow into a syringe to force him to strain properly. Didn't help. No amount of our coaching was working.

He really needed to get to the hospital, but he just wouldn't go. We were worried, but as long as he was not intoxicated and understood the risks he faced, we couldn't force him.

As time passed, we became more insistent that he was making a mistake, and he finally confessed.

"I can't go to the hospital because I'm not supposed to be here," he admitted.

"Okay, we get that, but this is confidential. Your boss won't find out you were here."

"No," he said, "I can't go to the hospital because my wife can't find out I was here."

Well, well...

We all looked at the young woman he was with and understood his plight. This could be a life-or-death situation on several levels. Finally, he curled himself into a ball with his knees to his chest and went to work, bearing down with the determination of a man facing divorce, or worse.

We were actually worried he might hurt himself. To our surprise, and luckily for him, it worked. His heart rate came down to a normal pace and he was able to rest for a while before returning to the festivities with his marriage intact. At least, for a while.

The vagal nerve starts in the brain as cranial nerve 10. It travels down the neck, chest, and abdomen and is part of the parasympathetic nervous system, which means it acts as a kind of brake and slows the heart rate when it's stimulated. You can also stimulate it by coughing forcefully or putting your face in cold water. Overstimulation, however, can cause fainting.

Part of my music festival "education" has been learning that people are people, no matter how they dress, what music they like, or how they behave. In the small town where I grew up, we didn't have much diversity. We all pretty much looked alike. Even getting your ears pierced was frowned upon.

As a father, I didn't allow my daughters to get tattoos or piercings other than in their ears. My professional colleagues were also conservatively dressed and generally had mainstream tastes. But I've been exposed to many people who don't look and dress like me now. Maybe they are covered in tattoos, have dreadlocks, or prefer a style of dress, or undress, that I wouldn't choose.

It has taken me a while, but as I've met and spoken to many who fit those descriptions, I've learned that they aren't much different than I am. The vast majority of them are nice, respectful people just trying to enjoy life. Not only did I find a new career, but I also discovered a new comfort zone.

Pink Tutu

I prefer to work out in the field at festivals and events rather than in the medical tent. I enjoy the adrenaline rush of responding to a scene, assessing the situation and the patient, and taking charge of that initial medical care. But there are experiences in the tent that have reminded me of the twists and turns my career has taken to carry me to this point.

The medical tent at this festival was divided into separate areas for critical and non-critical patients. I was working in the non-critical section. At many festivals, you see young ladies dressed in revealing clothes or even topless, but at this event there was full nudity among both men and women. Not a lot, but it wasn't uncommon to see people walking around with a hat, sunglasses, shoes, and nothing else. The vibe was relaxed to the point that the nudity almost went unnoticed. Almost.

On this particular day, attendees were encouraged to wear a tutu. When a couple came into the medical tent wearing pink tutus around their waists, we didn't think anything of it. Except that they appeared to be in their 70s, had urinary tract infections, and were totally naked but for the tutus. Without fanfare, the couple was led to my area where I helped the man onto a cot. A nurse asked me to start an IV on him so we could give him some fluid and get him hydrated. At that point in my career, I had not started many IVs and, though I was comfortable doing it, I was still a little nervous.

While I prepared everything, we had a pleasant conversation, as if he and his wife weren't stark naked wearing glittering, pink tutus. They had been to this festival many times, the man explained. He told me that he was retired, so I naturally asked him what he used to do.

"I was an emergency room doctor for 35 years."

I stopped what I was doing, looked at him, and said, "Oh great. Nothing like a little pressure to get this IV, right?"

Thankfully, he was extremely nice and had great veins.

As I cleaned the site and prepared to insert the IV catheter, it occurred to me that I was about to stick a needle in the arm of a very naked man as his equally naked, busty wife stood across the cot watching me work. I remember the moment clearly. The oddest part of it all? Neither they, nor I, were at all uncomfortable. It was as if I did this every day.

The IV went in with no trouble, the man and his wife were hydrated and given some antibiotics, and they left to enjoy the rest of the event. They were exceptionally thankful for our help and I was very happy to have met them. And to this day, it remains my only double-naked IV start.

Not all patients are so cooperative and grateful for our care. Some are downright hostile as my friend Sean reveals in the next story. In the beginning, I had no tolerance for this behavior. While many of my views have changed, my compassion still runs pretty low for jerks. The good news is, like in a casino, the house always wins and, in the end, patients get the medical care they need, even if they don't want it. Often, some well-deserved karma comes with it.

The Judge
As Told by Sean (Paramedic)

Very few things are as funny as a drunk concert-goer name-dropping when we are trying to take care of them. Their attempt to communicate their importance is far less intimidating when they slur their words and vomit on their shirt. The more they try, the funnier it becomes. And when it goes up the family chain, it becomes a story in this book.

I was working on the ambulance at a rap concert held near a local university. Because of its location, there were a lot of students and it was a very busy night. We made run after run, transporting patients to local hospitals. One of those patients was a student who was either drunk, high, or both – and he was being a serious ass. I don't know what brought him to the venue's medical room, but once there, he became my responsibility.

He tried his best to take charge of the situation and to let us know that he wasn't just some ordinary drunk college student. Oh no.

"You can't keep me here," he said. "You don't know who my father is."

"Okay, come on, buddy. You're going to the hospital."

"Fuck you, I'm not going anywhere."

Oh yes, he was. Because he was underage, we had no choice but to follow protocol and transport him. I didn't completely restrain him on our stretcher because I didn't want to make him angrier than he already was. But as we arrived at the hospital, he decided that he didn't like how things were going for him and took a swing at me. I grabbed him and pulled an arm behind his head to put him in the proper restraint position and brought him into the ER. Once in there, off-duty cops were in charge of combative patients, and I handed over Mr. Important.

"You'll be sorry when my dad gets here," the young man touted. "He's a judge. You're gonna be sorry."

None of us cared one bit about this underage smart-ass' father. We returned to the concert. He stayed in the ER firmly secured to his bed.

A few hours later, we brought another patient to that same ER. A friend of mine who worked there called me over.

"Hey Sean. That kid you brought in," my friend said. "His dad showed up."

"Oh, are we in trouble? He's a judge or something right?" I replied.

"Ha, no, you're not in trouble, but you'll want to see this."

She led me to the patient's room and opened the door. There, in the room together, were father and son, side by side, both in restraints, screaming, "You can't do this to us. You don't know who we are."

The Streaker

I was working the night shift at a music festival when we got a call to respond to the campground for multiple reports of a naked man shouting profanities. The reports of this foul-mouthed streaker came from different areas of the campground so we were unsure if there were several naked men or one very fast one. After a few minutes of driving around and interrogating campers, we found our solo exhibitionist. Security had him, and he was indeed naked.

They were struggling to subdue the young man, which isn't easy when your subject is naked and you need to be cautious about where you grab. Some of the medics I work with will jump into the fray and help security wrestle a hostile patient to the ground. I'm not one of them. I get enough bodily fluids on me in the normal course of events. Once security got him to the ground, I heroically hopped on one of his legs to keep him still enough for my partner to sedate him. The young man continued to squirm for a minute but eventually relented and calmed down.

"Hey, why are you guys being so rough with him? You don't need to hold him down."

It was a young woman in the crowd, watching and filming us with her phone.

"He was fighting security and we need to get him calmed down." I said.

"Yeah, but he tapped out."

I don't think I actually laughed aloud, at least I hope I didn't. An online video of me laughing at the situation would have looked bad.

"I'm recording everything you guys are doing to him," she said.

"Yeah fine, but maybe you could come help us instead?" I suggested.

That usually ends the conversation. And it did this time, too.

Our drug of choice for sedation at this festival was ketamine, a dissociative anesthetic, sedative, and painkiller. Ironically, even if the patient was running naked because he took ketamine recreationally, he got more ketamine. It acts quickly, doesn't depress the patient's respiratory function, and can even help keep blood pressure up. Now covered in dirt and grass, our naked man got a couple hundred milligrams of ketamine in his butt cheek and was taken to the medical tent – after we covered him with a blanket.

He wasn't the only naked patient that weekend. I was still a new EMT and this had me wondering, *Why do they get naked, and why only men?* We didn't have any calls for naked women screaming obscenities and the guys I saw streaking probably looked much better in clothes. So, it was odd to me that I was seeing these naked men.

I soon learned this: one reason people get naked at music festivals is because the drugs they've taken raise their temperatures until they're so hot they have to strip off their clothes to cool down. Subsequently, we sedate them to calm them down and lower their temperatures. So, if you see paramedics holding down a naked festival goer, it's not because we're abusive. It's because they need us to give them that shot of soothing "Special K" to cool down.

One of the dangers faced by festival goers is the use of impure or adulterated drugs. People who don't want to risk bringing drugs to the festival might buy them there from a stranger. There are several organizations that try to keep people safe by offering advice and providing them with kits to allow them to test the drugs. Those organizations are sometimes welcomed on-site at the festival, and sometimes are not, forcing them to do their work surreptitiously.

Bad Choices

We often run into "smart" attendees who don't want to risk being caught bringing drugs into the festival. Instead they get their supply from total strangers once through security and safely in the festival. Yeah, much smarter, right? At every festival, we meet a patient who took something that a stranger gave them and now didn't feel well.

Just recently I treated a patient who was in the crowd enjoying the music when a total stranger told him to open his mouth and stick out his tongue. He complied and the stranger put a small piece of paper on his tongue which then dissolved. A short time later, he saw me as I was walking across the grass toward our medical tent.

"Hey, are you medical?" he hollered.

Smart guy. My brightly colored shirt screamed "Medical" in large letters.

"Yes, I am. What's going on?"

"I don't feel well. I think I took something."

"What do you mean you *think* you took something?"

"Well, I was in the [mosh] pit and some guy told me to open my mouth and stick out my tongue. So, I did and he put a piece of paper on my tongue and it dissolved. Now I don't feel so good."

"Okay, well, have you ever used LSD before?"

"No, never."

"Well congratulations, you have now."

Dr. Jekyll
As Told by Jake (Paramedic)

I was assigned to the medical tent to help the nurses start IVs, take vital signs, and generally care for patients brought in from the stage areas. At this festival, the main medical tent was smaller with maybe 10 beds, and was staffed with paramedics, a nurse, and a resident doctor. One of our teams brought in a young woman who was seen in the crowd screaming at people and fighting. She was just generally disoriented. As I began my assessment, she remained both hostile and confused.

"Why am I here?" she asked.

"Because security saw you causing trouble in the crowd," I explained. "Why were you doing that?"

No answer.

"We want to make sure you're okay," I said.

"I don't want to be here. You can't make me." And with that, she stood up and ran out of the tent.

She didn't get far because security caught her and returned her to me. She tried to escape several more times, all without success. She alternated between crying, ranting, raving, and telling us that she was a doctor – an ophthalmologist, in fact. She believed this allowed her to tell us how we should treat her and when we should release her.

There also were times when she became quite friendly. Too friendly. When she wasn't running away, crying, or trying to assert her authority, she was trying to romance us. Several times she reached for me, rubbed my arms, and groped me in inappropriate places. She also groped another medic in the tent, so it wasn't just me. Perhaps it was a play for sympathy to let her go.

After about an hour, she again made a run for it, but this time ran right into the arms of a supervisor who was big enough to grab her. Frustrated by this, she proceeded to bite the supervisor in his arm to the point of drawing blood.

That's all it took. She had finally found a way to escape.

Four police officers who had witnessed the entire episode handcuffed her and escorted her out of the medical tent to the local jail.

A number of years ago, my wife and I hosted a holiday party. We had 20 or so friends in our home, eating and chatting, when my college-age daughter came downstairs to go out with some friends. She was wearing a very short skirt, spike heels, and some type of blouse that I thought was all too revealing.

I had the ultimate Dad moment when I asked, "Is that what you're wearing out?"

She looked lovely, but it made me uncomfortable. By music festival standards, she was well covered up, but she was my *daughter*.

Since then, I've become almost immune to seeing young women, and men, barely dressed. I sometimes wonder if the goal is to see how little they can wear and still say they are wearing something. I've also learned that I'm not the only parent who is uncomfortable with some fashion choices. My paramedic friend Jerone is too.

Mom's Revenge
As Told by Jerone (Paramedic)

Showcasing fashion at a music festival, in particular EDM festivals, seems to be an affair unto itself. Particularly for young women, clothing is often skimpy, sometimes sheer, and occasionally missing. In fact, *Elle* magazine published a Festival Fashion Guide in 2019 for its readers to be sure they had the right look. For parents of these young women, however, it can be eye-opening.

A young woman of perhaps 19 was brought into the medical tent and was either high, very intoxicated, or both. That wasn't unusual, but what she wore was striking. She had black tape Xs covering her nipples, a pink tutu around her waist, a white thong, and UGG boots. That was it.

We placed her on a cot, did our usual assessment, and started an IV to rehydrate her. I was able to get her information from the chip in her festival bracelet and saw that she was indeed underage. That meant an automatic call to her parents.

"Hello, ma'am. I'm a paramedic working in the medical tent at [the music festival] and we have your daughter here," I said. "She's okay, but someone will need to come pick her up or we will have to transport her to the hospital."

"Who is this? Is this a joke? You have the wrong number," said the woman who had answered the phone.

"Ma'am, is your daughter Mary Smith?" I asked.

"Yes, but she's not at any music festival. Who is this really?"

"As I said, Mrs. Smith, I'm a paramedic and I am at [the festival] in the medical tent with your daughter."

"I don't know what you think you are doing, but my daughter is next door at a friend's house," the woman argued.

"No ma'am, she is here in my medical tent. You need to come get her and you should bring some clothes for her."

"Honey!" she called to her husband. "Some guy is on the phone saying he is with Mary in a medical tent. Go next door and make sure she's there."

I waited as I heard her husband leave the house and return a few minutes later. I heard muffled conversation in the background. Suddenly the woman, Mary's mother, was contrite.

"I'll be right there," she said.

I added, "And bring some clothes."

A short time later, I met Mary's mother at the entrance to our tent. She was understandably angry and concerned. By then, her daughter had sobered up enough to leave with a parent, so we released her. As she walked from her cot to her mom, she never looked up, staring at the floor the whole way. When she reached the entrance, she asked her mom, "Can I have some clothes, please?"

"Absolutely not," her mother said, "You're going home like that so your father can see how you are dressed."

Oh my God, I thought. *That is going to be one uncomfortable ride home.*

My first concert was Linda Ronstadt at an outdoor pavilion in northeast Ohio. I've been to many more, but all fall into a pretty tight genre of "old people rock n' roll." As a paramedic, I've worked festivals and concerts of all types: The Rolling Stones, Taylor Swift, and BTS K-Pop, to name a few. I loved the Stones, enjoyed Coldplay, hated Kiss, and was intrigued by BTS.

Surprisingly, EDM festivals have become my favorite. Yes, you read that correctly. This old stodgy, starched-shirt lawyer likes EDM. In addition to the unique vibe, EDM concert-goers are generally not throwing up on us and are most often pleasant and happy. I attribute that to less alcohol, more drugs.

In the EDM culture, drug use seems intended to enhance the musical experience and to give the user energy. Other festivals and concerts seem to foster drinking just to get drunk, which leads to a very different patient experience. People who have overdone their party drugs may be wild and out of control, but I can safely sedate them so they become docile and go to sleep. Patients who have had too much to drink are often passed out and either have, or soon will, vomit. They can also be more hostile.

This is a pretty sweeping generalization, but I think most medical professionals who have worked these events will agree. My views have changed as I have experienced both, but I speak only from the standpoint of taking care of the people who need help, not as someone who endorses recreational drug use and alcohol. As a paramedic and a father, my hope is that if you drink or take drugs, you do it safely and responsibly.

Planet Earth

I am often asked if I use a lot of Narcan, which was created to block the effect of opioids, when I work at these festivals. The answer is no. I've given it twice, both times because we were unsure what was going on with the patient. The opioid crisis has brought Narcan to the general public's attention and it's an amazing drug when needed. However, it's used to reverse the effects of narcotics like heroin or fentanyl which are "downers." Drugs at music festivals tend to be "uppers" that make people happy and energetic. Fortunately, we don't see frequent narcotic use or have to deal with overdoses.

That's why I wasn't too concerned when I met a young man at a festival sitting on the ground with a variety of pills spread out in front of him. He was in an area with portable lockers where attendees could lock their valuables while they enjoyed the shows. He sat cross-legged and moved several dozen pills around on the ground. It looked random to me, or at least I couldn't see what he was trying to do, but I greeted him as I usually do.

"Hi sir, what's going on?" I asked.

"Nothing." He didn't look up at me but continued shuffling his pills.

"My name is Jim. What's yours?"

"Steven." So far, so good.

"Steven, do you know where you are?" I asked.

"Yes."

"Where are you?"

He hesitated a moment before slowly saying, "I… am on… the planet… Earth."

My partner laughed behind me. "He's not wrong."

Oriented as to place – check.

Of course, digging a little deeper made it clear that Steven most definitely did not know where on our beautiful planet he was at the moment, so we guided him onto the cart for a ride to the medical tent. My partner rode with the crew, worried that Steven's calm behavior may change. He was right.

When Steven saw the row of ambulances and his new reality set in, he became violent and needed several security guards and paramedics to subdue and sedate him for a trip to a different part of Earth – the ER.

———

Paramedics conduct a primary assessment as soon as they meet a patient. In short, it consists of checking the patient's mental status (Are they alert, responsive to voice or pain, or unresponsive?), whether their airway is open, whether they are breathing, and whether they have a pulse. The goal is to find any immediate life threats and fix them. Only then do paramedics move on to a more detailed assessment of the patient. In the case of Steven, I knew his airway was open and he was breathing as soon as he spoke to me. And no sign of bleeding meant he didn't have any immediate life threats that we could fix.

———

IT'S NOT ALL FUN AND GAMES, IS IT?

"What we have once enjoyed deeply, we can never lose. All that we love deeply becomes a part of us." – Helen Keller

Summer 2018, I worked at a Taylor Swift concert at Soldier Field in Chicago. I was assigned to a team on the floor next to the stage. Like most well-known artists, Ms. Swift had a litany of private security. The man in charge of her team introduced himself, brought us up on stage, and gave us a general briefing about what they would do if there were any security or safety problems. He also showed us his "mass casualty" box which contained tourniquets, pressure bandages, and vented seals for penetrating wounds to the chest.

I was impressed with his professional demeanor and his preparedness. But always one to ask dumb questions, I said, "That's great to be so prepared, but you're just being super cautious, right? You don't really expect to need all of that stuff?"

He stopped walking, turned to me, and said as nicely as he could, "Nobody remembers the Jason Aldean concert in Vegas for the music." Ouch.

He was right, of course. The tragic events in Las Vegas in October 2017 began as just an ordinary show to conclude a weekend music festival and ended with 58 people dead and more than 400 wounded. It was not the first such mass tragedy at a concert and probably wouldn't be the last. Bad things can and do happen on a smaller scale, and they are just as tragic for those involved.

These are the calls that test and scare us, but for which we have prepared and trained. These are the calls, I have learned, that separate what we do from almost any other job. These are also the calls that can haunt us. Often, the difference between life and death is how close the person is to a medical resource or whether their friends are capable of alerting someone to help. In those moments, the fun stops and our real work begins.

The Fall
As Told by Pam (Paramedic) and John (Paramedic)

Pam: I was working in dispatch at a local festival that took place in a large parking lot surrounding a sports stadium. There were stages both inside the stadium and outside in the parking lots. I was in the command center with dispatchers for security, housekeeping, and customer relations. The room was small enough that we could speak easily to each other and pass along information.

It was late afternoon when the security dispatcher took a call from one of their people saying that a patron had fallen outside their window. As she was talking to the caller, I could see a look of horror appear on her face as she learned the person had fallen from a high height to the ground. She quickly shared the information with me and I radioed the closest mobile team. I wasn't sure what to expect, but it was clear this was not a typical kind of call.

John: I was assigned to the transport cart at the festival with a new EMT partner. It had been a pretty typical day for a festival like this, so when we got a call that someone had fallen, I didn't think too much about it. We were perhaps a quarter of the way around the outside of the stadium from where the fall had happened, so it took us a couple minutes to make our way through the crowd, even on a cart with lights and a siren. When we arrived, our expectations of a routine call changed rapidly.

In front of us was a young man, probably in his twenties, lying on his back on the cement walkway next to the outside wall of the stadium. He was not moving; we could see he had severe head injuries. We later learned that he had been inside the stadium waiting on a friend to use the bathroom. He had decided to sit on the outside wall of the stadium ramp which was waist-high. As he had attempted to light a cigarette, he had leaned back and fallen over the wall about 30 feet to the ground. He had landed directly on his back.

Even as we pulled up to the scene, we could see that not only was his head bleeding, but it was severely deformed. Because I had been a paramedic for many years and had seen too many head traumas to count, I immediately recognized that this young man was unlikely to survive these injuries. Our supervisor arrived at about the same time and went to the young man. He reached and felt along the side of his neck.

"No pulse, let's go!" he barked.

At this point, we went into full cardiac arrest mode, notified our ambulance to come immediately, and began CPR on the patient. He was obviously not breathing, but an enormous amount of bleeding prevented me from intubating him. We began to suction his airway and ventilate him with our bag-valve mask as best we could. Another team showed up and placed the AED pads on his chest, but the AED determined that no shock was advised. I was not surprised. There was not enough electrical activity in his heart to benefit from a shock.

At some point, I became aware that people in the VIP boxes above the scene were watching us, including politicians from the town hosting the festival. A crowd of spectators had gathered around us. I remember feeling like we were putting on a show for everyone.

While it seemed longer, we worked on him for only a few minutes when our ambulance arrived. By then, I had secured an IV in his arm so the ambulance medics could give him drugs and fluids if necessary. As we continued to perform CPR, the AED maintained that no shock was advised. We loaded him into the ambulance, turning over his care to the paramedics who took him to the nearest ER. I was left with my partner, a pool of blood, plastic wrappers from our equipment, and a group of stunned onlookers.

Sadly, none of our hard work mattered. The young man did not survive. He was just an ordinary guy out with his friends for a day of fun at a music festival. I had done all I could to save him, but it hadn't been enough. That's the hardest part of our job.

I was later told that the mayor and other VIPs were impressed by our response and efforts to save the young man's life.

It was no comfort to me.

His parents were about to get the worst phone call of their lives.

Bleeding Out
As Told by Josh (Paramedic)

I typically work the day shift at music festivals for the simple reason that I love the music and want to enjoy the shows at night. On the opening day of this particular festival, people were coming into the campgrounds or just waking up in their tents. It was a pretty typical summer day in the Midwest, cool but heating up with bright sunshine and dew soaking the grass. My team was dispatched to the campground for a reported syncopal event, which meant someone had fainted. These types of calls vary from something pretty serious like a cardiac problem to someone who was a little dehydrated and stood up too fast, so I really didn't know what to expect.

When we found the patient, he was sitting upright on the back of his friend's SUV with the rear door open. My first observation was that he didn't look good. He was very pale and his skin was cool and sweaty. But we could discern nothing to explain his appearance. His friends told us that he had just passed out and woken up shortly afterwards, but I didn't see anything that would lead me to think he had a seizure. He had no history of falls or any recent trauma or head injury. And they insisted he hadn't taken any drugs. The only thing I noticed was a small drop of blood on his gym shorts, but I didn't think too much of it. There was no sign of bleeding anywhere else.

Obviously, we wanted to take him to the main medical area to be fully evaluated, but when my partner and I grabbed under his shoulders and stood him up, we saw a very large volume of blood begin to flow freely from his anus. That changed everything. We quickly laid him down on the ground and again quizzed his friends.

"Okay guys, what's the deal? What's he been doing?" I asked, now very concerned.

His girlfriend stepped in. "You know what? He had a colonoscopy yesterday," she said. "Could that be it?"

Yes, that most definitely could be it. My partner and I were now in full assess-and-treat mode.

"Joe, get another blood pressure. I'm getting an IV." As I grabbed my supplies, I heard my partner's voice.

"Crap, he is 60 over palp."

This now explained his symptoms – his fainting, his cool but sweaty skin, and his pale complexion. A blood pressure reading below 90 is concerning; one that is 60 is dangerously low. And with that much bleeding, he was in hypovolemic shock. Even as an experienced paramedic, seeing that much blood and hearing his BP number was a holy-crap moment. This wasn't in someone's home or the back of an ambulance. We were in the middle of a field in a remote town dealing primarily with healthy, young adults. Having a patient bleed out on me was not something I had expected to see that weekend.

I started a large IV in his arm and connected a bag of saline to it. He needed fluid replacement in a hurry. As we transported him to the medical tent, I called ahead to alert the staff he was going to need an ambulance immediately. When we arrived, the doctor looked at him, quickly took another set of vital signs, and agreed that he needed an ER right away. Because there are always ambulances on standby at the medical tent, within minutes of arriving, he was on his way to a hospital with top-notch medics caring for him on the trip. As for me, I spent the next hour cleaning his blood off of me, changing my clothes, disinfecting our equipment, and doing paperwork. I wrote a very detailed report of the incident, expecting it to go to a lawyer at some point.

This was a memorable call, but there are two things that have really stayed in my mind. First, I remember how badly the patient felt for his friends. He apologized to them repeatedly as we were tried to get him loaded into our cart. He was much more concerned that he was ruining the festival for them than he was concerned for himself. And as thoughtful as that was, he really needed to get to the ER. The second thing I can't get out of my head is the scene itself. The smell was horrific and, even though we were not there long, the flies descended within minutes to crawl all over the blood. Even talking about it now makes me want to go take a long shower.

People often describe someone as going into shock when they are shaken up or look pale and sweaty. For paramedics, shock is a physiological condition in which the person stops perfusing, meaning there is not enough blood circulating, or air going in and out, to keep cells alive. In other words, something has caused your blood pressure to drop and your blood isn't moving through your arteries and veins like it should. This deprives your cells of oxygen, and bad things begin to happen.

Brain Bleed
As Told by Nathan (EMT)

My partner and I were assigned to be outside on our medical cart as the crowd arrived for a big event. It was colder than normal and most people were dressed for it. Based on what I was seeing, I suspected they had also been drinking to stay warm. Dispatch called and told us to respond to the parking garage for an unknown reason. It's unusual for dispatch not to have *some* information about a call, even if it turns out to be incorrect, so we were a little skeptical. We expected someone who really didn't need our help. We were wrong.

We found a young man in his twenties lying unconscious at the bottom of a set of stairs that led from the top deck of the parking garage. Draped over the last step, he was unmoving with blood pooling around his head. He did not acknowledge our voices and barely flinched in response to a painful stimulus.

Paramedics and doctors use the Glasgow Coma Score to assess someone's level of consciousness which helps determine the severity of an injury. It measures responsiveness in terms of opening their eyes, and their ability to speak, and follow commands. A healthy adult is a GCS of 15 out of 15. The lowest possible score a patient can receive is a 3. This patient was a 6.

We immediately stabilized his neck and spine with a cervical collar and put pressure against the site of the bleeding. My partner called dispatch.

"Dispatch from Team 8."

"Go ahead, Team 8."

"We need the ambo here immediately for a trauma. Patient is unresponsive."

"Are you doing CPR, Team 8?"

"Negative, patient has a pulse and is breathing on his own right now."

We carefully moved him to our backboard, put him on our cart, and drove to the other end of the parking deck to meet the ambulance. On the crew that day were two very experienced paramedics who went right to work. As we loaded the backboard onto their stretcher, the young man stopped breathing and began posturing involuntarily, a dangerous sign of brain trauma. He clenched his teeth tightly so we could not intubate him without administering drugs, a process that wasn't in our protocols.

He was bleeding out of his ears, a sign of a possible skull fracture, which meant we could not put an airway in his nostrils to help deliver oxygen to him. Inserting a nasal airway can kill a patient in that situation. We had to bag him the best we could to get much-needed oxygen into his lungs and to his brain. He was also starting to show signs of brain herniation, a condition characterized by the swelling of the brain. Since the pressure has no way to escape, it forces the brain down through the base of the skull quite often killing the victim. His blood pressure was in the 180s and his heart rate was in the 40s. Those are two of the three signs of Cushing's Triad, a lethal set of symptoms.

Once in the ambulance and heading to the nearest trauma center, we began to cut his clothes off so we could fully assess him. Had he incurred any additional injuries? It turned out that he was well-prepared for the cold weather. We cut off multiple layers of shirts and pants. We had shredded clothes all over the ambulance. In removing his clothes, we discovered that the patient had an involuntary erection called priapism, another sign of significant head or spine trauma.

When we arrived at the trauma center, the surgeon met us and was able to intubate the young man immediately. He was x-rayed and taken to surgery right away. We later learned two things about the patient – one surprised us, the other didn't. We were told that the young man had a blood alcohol level five times the legal limit. This was at 11 a.m., well before the event had started.

We also learned that, despite a skull fracture and two areas of bleeding in his brain, he recovered fully and walked out of the hospital several weeks later.

I don't know if our efforts made the difference in his recovery, but I do know that this lucky young man received excellent pre-hospital care, and I was very proud to have been part of the team that had provided it.

The Save
As Told by Jon (EMT)

In a pre-hospital setting like a music festival, a "save" is generally used to describe a response to a cardiac arrest patient whom we resuscitate and bring back to life. It can also be used to describe other severely critical patients who are stabilized by paramedics, allowing them to get to the hospital and survive serious injuries or illness. These "saves" happen infrequently for EMTs and paramedics, but when they do, they are amazing. It is usually because things worked exactly as they were supposed to, even in the midst of chaos.

I was at a concert in the VIP section with a female patient who was vomiting. As we were about to take her to the first aid room, I received a call over my radio of a cardiac arrest outside the venue and was told to proceed there immediately. There were other medical personnel with the woman, so I left. I was not far and was able to get to the second patient quickly.

When I arrived, another medic and an EMT were already there doing chest compressions on a young woman and preparing to intubate her so we could give oxygen directly into her lungs. The patient, who was maybe in her late thirties, had been working at a vendor booth when she had suddenly collapsed. Her co-workers had called for help right away and our team had responded quickly. Good-quality CPR had started within a few minutes of her collapse.

I had taken over chest compressions while the other EMT began to put the defibrillation pads on her chest when I noticed one of her fingers begin to move and her eyelids flicker. We did a quick check and found she now had a pulse, but she was still not breathing on her own. The medic finished the intubation and we started to breathe for her. By then, the ambulance had arrived, so we moved her to the stretcher; they continued her care as they transported her to a hospital equipped to treat cardiac emergencies.

I later learned that the woman had a history of pulmonary embolisms, or blood clots, in her lungs, and had suffered one that day. These clots block the forward flow of blood coming from the heart preventing them from being oxygenated in the lungs. That blockage causes the heart to have to work harder to deliver blood to the lungs. Depending on the severity, it can sometimes cause the heart to stop.

Fortunately, this patient received prompt treatment to remove the clots and recovered well. Her good fortune was largely due to the chain of survival that had been seamlessly implemented. There was an immediate call for help, prompt, high-quality CPR, quick transportation to an appropriate facility, and proper treatment at the hospital.

Someone had been watching over her, and us, that day.

It was a reminder why everyone should get trained in CPR. It's easy and dramatically increases the odds of a person surviving a devastating event.

When a person goes into cardiac arrest, the single best response is immediate chest compressions at a rate of 100 to 120 per minute. There is no need to breathe for them until EMS arrives. Press hard and fast on the center of the chest to the beat of "Stayin' Alive" by the Bee Gees. Don't be afraid to hurt the person; they are dead. And without immediate CPR, they are likely to stay that way. Studies show that bystander CPR can double or triple the chance of survival.

OMG! THAT'S DISGUSTING

"Well, they can't prove whose vomit it was…You can't really dust for vomit."
– This is Spinal Tap

When people learn that I am a paramedic, they quite often get an odd look on their faces, as if they are smelling a noxious odor. They say, "I could never do that. I can't stand to see blood." At music festivals, the truth is that blood is not the most common bodily fluid we encounter. Depending on the type of music, varying levels of alcohol intoxication are present; with alcohol comes vomit. Sometimes, lots of it. Less-experienced drinkers excited by their surroundings often overdo it to the point of passing out. And when you are passed out, you don't have control of your bodily functions. In those cases, I would be much happier dealing with a little blood.

Two of the staples in the medical tent at many music festivals are absorbent sawdust and disposable cardboard buckets, the kind

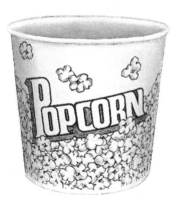

you get at the movie theater when you buy a large popcorn. They are round with a big opening, made of solid construction, and have a flat bottom. They are perfect for catching vomit. No need to clean it out; just throw it away. Depending on how hot it is on a given festival day which influences how much people may drink, we can go through hundreds of these buckets.

When a patient is brought in with any potential to be sick – which is most of them – we automatically give them a bucket with instructions on how to use it. That should be pretty self-explanatory, but all too often, we see patients lying on army-style cots, feeling the urge, and leaning over the edge of the cot to throw up on the floor while the popcorn bucket sits empty on their lap. That's where the absorbent sawdust comes in. By the end of the night, it is piled up in between the cots waiting to be shoveled into the trash bins. It's so prevalent that it goes largely unnoticed by those of us caring for patients.

One patient, a young man who was perhaps in his mid-twenties, impressed us with his understanding of the popcorn bucket process, at least for a while. I hadn't seen this patient be brought in nor did I know his condition. A lot goes on in these medical tents with so many moving parts, so it's not uncommon to suddenly notice someone new lying on a cot.

When I first saw him, he was sitting up on the cot with his legs crossed in front of him. He had on shorts and a white T-shirt. He was a nice-looking young man and seemed pretty aware of his surroundings. He had been given a popcorn bucket, which told me several things: he had been checked in, his vital signs had been taken, and someone had thought he might throw up. Whoever that person was got it right.

I decided to check on him.

"Hey buddy, you doing okay?" I asked.

"Yeah, I'm cool."

"I see you have your bucket. Can I get you anything else?"

"Nah, I'm cool," he said.

I was standing nearby, talking to one of the resident doctors working there when Mr. Cool grabbed the bucket, leaned forward, and vomited profusely. Amazingly, the contents of his stomach went entirely into the bucket. It appeared not a drop went astray. I think I actually exclaimed my amazement aloud, or perhaps it just seemed that way. It was an unusual degree of success I had just witnessed.

Unfortunately, my celebration was premature. The young man picked up the bucket filled with his vomit and turned it upside down, pouring the contents all over his lap and onto the floor.

Good grief. More sawdust, please.

This took place on my second night at a music festival, the day after I saved the life of the woman on her cell phone with her mom. For others, this young man's action was no big deal. To me, it was shocking. I went home and told my wife that if people want to educate their kids on the dangers of alcohol, the medical tent is the place to be. *Holy crap, what a mess*, I thought.

With time though, I have come to love the medical tent. It is an assortment of life and personalities that I don't think exists anywhere else.

I was discussing my medical tent experiences with a friend who has worked in them for many years and I shared the popcorn bucket story with him.

His response?

Hold my beer.

Tastes Great
As Told by Jerone (Paramedic)

A young woman came into the medical tent with one of our field teams. She was young, in her early-twenties. I was told she was a little too rambunctious out in the festival area. Our sense was she had a combination of Molly and alcohol on board. We put her on a cot next to a young man who had also enjoyed his Molly a little too much and needed to ride it out with us. I remember her asking for water, getting water, and then falling asleep on her cot, spilling it. This happened several times, so we decided to allow her no more water. Between her naps, she and her cot neighbor got to know each other. I saw them several times reach across the space between the cots and touch each other in the way only those on Molly can: gently, compassionately, romantically.

At one point, she indicated she was feeling nauseous, so we gave her one of our ever-present popcorn buckets in case she vomited. She again asked for water but was told that it would be best not to drink anything. Her newfound friend, feeling generous, eagerly shared his water with her. She took a long drink and promptly vomited into the bucket. Normally, this barely registered with us because so many of our patients were doing it. As long as they were not at risk of choking, we simply allowed them to get it out of their systems.

This time though, I happened to be looking at our patient as she grasped the bucket with both hands, brought it up to her mouth, tipped it, and took a sip. From the bucket.

"What the hell are you doing?" I yelled, darting toward her.

"Nothin." And then she did it again, this time taking a gulp, and then another, of her own vomit.

God damn. What was she doing?

And then she started to seize. Full on, convulsive seizure. On the cot, puke and all.

Another medic was nearby and came right over. Seizures are always dangerous. But in circumstances like this when drugs may be in someone's system, it can be even more of an emergency. And I knew nothing about this patient's history. We immediately began looking for a place to start an IV, but she had really poor veins. I had been a medic for a long time, so my go-to solution when that happened was to start an IV in the external jugular vein of the patient's neck. I was able to get it in and hooked up to some saline quickly. We also gave her some Midazolam to stop her seizures. We discovered later that she had a history of epilepsy so, as we suspected, her seizure was unrelated to her choice of drink at that moment.

We shipped her off to an ER to allow them to continue her care. The story of the girl who drank her own vomit became legendary and is retold every year as new EMTs and medics join us in the tent.

Patients who are so intoxicated or high that they are not aware enough to turn their head if they get sick present a serious risk of choking on their vomit and inhaling it into their lungs. This can cause serious pneumonia and other significant respiratory problems. They require a higher level of oversight and care than we can usually provide in a medical tent. We transport them to an ER to be sure they receive appropriate care.

As I re-read these stories now, it feels all too normal. Just another day at the office. The shock value has diminished. That in and of itself is shocking. Never would I have imagined myself in these situations. Yet three years into my festival medic career, I simply shrug and acknowledge that yes, I've been there, done that, and have the stains on my pants to prove it.

Trippin' Balls
As Told by Jerone (Paramedic)

When a person takes drugs that firmly controls their mind and body, they are said to be "trippin' balls." I know this because of my work in the medical tents at various festivals, not because I do the trippin' myself. Every year, I see at least one patient who is severely under the influence and quite often will announce their ball-trippin' status to me.

The young man in this story walked into our tent on his own, a pretty admirable feat given he was clearly lost in a drug-induced fog. I remember him because he was wearing one of the greatest Panama hats I'd ever seen. In addition to the cool hat, he was wearing proper khaki shorts and a preppy polo shirt. That made him well-dressed by festival standards; by his own admission, he was high on Molly and ketamine. I've learned these kids will start with some Molly to get things rolling, then add a "bump" of ketamine and possibly more later.

This young man didn't need more; he needed a nap. Or at least that's what he told us. So, we led him to a cot, checked his vital signs, and let him lay down to sleep it off.

"I need to make a phone call first," he said.

"Sorry, but you can't use a phone in here," I replied.

"No, it's okay," he told us. "You won't be able to see it."

Well, that got my attention. I was curious and went to his cot to see what he had in mind. I watched as he pulled a regular water bottle out of his pocket and proceeded to "dial" numbers on the side of it. He then held it to the side of his head and began a conversation with his friend, who I guess also had a water-bottle phone. I listened as he told his imaginary friend that he needed to hang up because he had to use the bathroom. He promised to call him back.

What I didn't realize until a few minutes later is that he did not need to go to the bathroom. Oh no. While on the phone, speaking to his friend, he had defecated and urinated all over himself and our cot. We discovered this when he began to complain about the smell – his smell. He then vomited on himself and the person in the cot next to him. Yes, a real medical-tent star he was. We promptly packaged this kid up and loaded him into an ambulance heading to the ER. I am sure the nurses were quite happy to receive him.

Festival Fail

The mood at these music festivals is always high-spirited. People are with friends and having fun. It's no secret that some of the patrons consume alcohol and use party drugs, sometimes to an extreme. The producers of the festivals are very strict about underage drinking. To buy alcohol in most festival grounds, you need a wristband obtainable only with ID. But they can't control what happens outside the gate before the show. And at one of my festivals, there is a common practice of pre-gaming – drinking on the way to the festival or after you get there but before the gates open. This particular year, it cost several young ladies a great day of music.

The gates had not yet opened; I believe it was around 10:30 a.m. when my partner and I got a call to go to the main entrance for a "sick" person outside the gate. When we arrived, we found a small group of young women, age unknown, gathered around their friend who was sitting on the sidewalk with her back to a cement barricade. Her head was in her hands and she was not very responsive when we attempted to talk to her. As I recall, she mostly just moaned.

My partner began to question her friends.

"Has she been drinking?" he asked.

One of her friends jumped in. "Yeah, on the train coming in we had some stuff to drink."

"How much did she have?"

"I'm not sure, but maybe too much."

You think?

As we always do, we checked the woman's vital signs. Other than appearing to be very intoxicated, we had no reason to be concerned. One of the ladies told us that her dad was on his way to pick them up and take them home, but with street closures, he was unsure where to meet us. So, we agreed to walk with them a couple blocks up the main thoroughfare to make it easier for Dad. We were able to get the young lady up to her feet and moving forward, but she was pretty wobbly. It didn't help that the sidewalks were crowded with festival goers arriving and others simple walking to or from work.

We had reached an intersection and were waiting for the light to turn in our favor when the young woman, who I was supporting, said calmly, "Oooh" and then bent over and threw up on my shoes and pants, and all over the city street corner. The crowd of people waiting to cross the street dispersed quickly as the light changed.

At that point, three things became clear to me: 1. the young lady had not eaten in some time; 2. the young lady had had quite a bit to drink; and 3. I was very glad the young lady was not getting into my car.

We managed to meet her friend's dad who fortuitously had a blanket in the trunk of his car. After spreading it on the back seat, we loaded her into the car with her friends and watched as they drove off.

I don't know how far they had to drive or how long it took in traffic. I was unsure if there was anything at all left in the young woman's stomach. But I was sure that it was not going to be a pleasant trip home.

Seeing Red

Not long ago during my training, I asked an experienced paramedic when he finally felt like he knew what was going on and how to deal with it. I expected him to tell me it took a couple years. His response was that he would let me know if he ever felt that way, because every call ultimately could be something he had yet to see. That was both terrifying and exhilarating. I don't like the feeling of not being fully confident, yet constantly learning and being challenged with new things provides the intellectual stimulation I enjoy. I have seen and learned quite a bit in three years, but the more I learn, the more I realize how much I don't know.

We rarely deal with blood at these events, but there are exceptions. I was still new to the event scene when I worked at a concert in a large stadium. About the only difference between a concert and a festival is that we generally get to transport our patients across concrete floors instead of grass, dirt, and rocks. The area we cover is generally smaller as well, so help can often arrive more quickly when you need it. That comes in handy for patients with serious issues.

At this event, I was assigned to a field team with my partner and given a location to report to when available for a call. Well, before the show began, as fans were just coming in, dispatch called and told my partner and I to respond to one of the concessions stands for a report of a person bleeding. That was the extent of the information.

We were on the concrete concourse that led around the inside of the stadium. We had our medical bags on our stair chair and a folding metal chair with wheels, which is how we transport patients at many events. After walking about 30 yards, we saw a small pool of blood on the floor, which turned into a steady crimson trail. We were pretty sure we were on the right path, so to speak.

At about this time, our supervisor called us on the radio. "Team 2, I'm with the patient. What's your ETA to me?"

"We are about 30 seconds away," I responded.

"Hurry up and get your gloves on."

While we always wear gloves as part of our protection, it's unusual to be instructed to get them on before we arrive. The sense of urgency in our supervisor's voice also unnerved me.

When we got to the patient's location, we understood his concern. We found our supervisor applying pressure to the bloodied calf of a middle-aged man. On the floor around him was an alarming pool of blood. Because I had my gloves on, I offered to take my supervisor's place. As he released his grip, a thin stream of blood shot from the side of the patient's leg about 10 feet across the concourse and continued to flow. I didn't expect such forceful bleeding. I immediately grabbed his calf and put pressure on the wound, which was just a tiny pinprick along the outside of his leg. I had seen a lot of bleeding wounds, but I had never seen one with forceful spurting like that. And the amount of blood on the floor was significant.

"Is this arterial?" I asked the boss. Arterial bleeds are usually the ones under high pressure.

"No," he said, "Ruptured varicose vein." Interesting.

I knew about varicose veins, of course, but had never heard of them rupturing and bleeding like that. I was now close-up familiar with it.

Apparently, this gentleman had been standing at an ATM getting cash when a woman had approached him and told him his leg was bleeding. That was the first indication to him that something was amiss. Someone had called in to dispatch, which is what had gotten the ball rolling. The gentleman had pulled up the leg of his jeans and began to walk toward our first aid room, leaving a trail of blood for us to discover. The supervisor had come from the other direction, saw him, and grabbed hold of his calf to stop the flow of blood. That's when he had called us.

We were able to wrap his leg with gauze tight enough to stop the bleeding as we took him to our first aid room. There we took his vital signs and saw that his blood pressure was extremely high. As I recall, his systolic (top number) was well over 200 and his diastolic (bottom number) was over 100. Other than being anxious about what was going on, the man said he felt fine. Obviously, though, he needed to be seen in an ER and was quickly transported by ambulance.

I have since learned that ruptured varicose veins like this are a fairly common life-threatening emergency. Fortunately for this man, he was in a place where he got immediate high-quality medical attention and was in an emergency room in less than 45 minutes.

When you hear your blood pressure, the top number (systolic) is the pressure of blood passing through your arteries during a heartbeat. The bottom number (diastolic) is the pressure during the brief pause between heartbeats. If your pressure is too low, not enough blood and the oxygen it carries will get to important organs, like your brain. If your pressure is too high, it can damage the arteries and lead to stroke or cardiac issues.

ARE THEY ALL THIS FRISKY?

"If you can't be with the one you love…love the one you're with." – Stephen Stills

I've mentioned a few times so far that the mood at these festivals is almost always entirely upbeat and friendly. People are happy, giving lots of hugs, and at night in the campgrounds, well, you can imagine. But that friendliness can sometimes cross the line.

You may remember that the drug Molly releases dopamine, norepinephrine, and serotonin in your brain. Serotonin is a feel-good hormone that can elevate your mood and cause you to feel closeness and empathy for a person. In the extreme, it can cause you to want to be extremely close to a person, even a stranger. Occasionally, we are those strangers.

I have never taken Molly and had never been around anyone who had until I became a paramedic. My first exposure to it was with a patient we transported to the ER. I first saw him on a chair in our medical tent quietly watching what was going on. It's unusual to see a patient just sitting there, so I went and talked to him. He was a nice young guy, but I noticed right away that his pupils were dilated, almost to the point of eliminating the colored part of his eye. That was a big tip off that he was on some stimulant, and, in this case, most likely Molly.

We were going to be taking an extremely intoxicated young woman to the ER and so decided to take him as well. She remained passed out on our stretcher while he sat in our jump seat in the ambulance. It was just a 10-minute ride to the hospital, but he was very concerned for the young woman's welfare the entire time. He asked repeatedly if she was going to be okay. He couldn't take his eyes off her, not in a creepy way, but in a concerned, caring way. It was both sweet and funny at the same time. I had yet to learn how this symptom could go into overdrive and produce some hilarious, if inappropriate, situations.

Pleasure Cruise

Our company had been hired to provide medical support for a medium-sized EDM festival. It was early in the season and one of the first festivals of the year. My partner and I were assigned to one of two specialized golf carts used to transport patients from the scene or from smaller medical tents to the main tent. These carts had room in the back for a backboard and a seat next to it along with our medical bags. They were perfect for transporting patients with flashing lights and a siren to alert people that an emergency vehicle was coming through. They also had a plastic windshield to keep the dust out of our eyes as we drove along dirt paths.

We had just brought a patient to the main medical tent when we heard the second transport team report over our radio that they had a patient who needed to go straight out to the hospital. In the background, we heard their patient screaming as they were being transported. I recall that everyone stopped and looked at each other. *Probably a hostile patient who was not happy about going to medical*, I thought, hearing the patient making all kinds of ruckus in the background. I could only imagine the difficulty my colleagues were having trying to control this unruly woman. As you may have guessed by now, this story takes an unusual turn. So, I'll let Nathan, the EMT who cared for the patient, take it from here.

As Told by Nathan (EMT)

We heard several reports from one of our satellite medical tents that they had a combative patient. No one was responding to the radio calls, so we drove off as safely as we could to provide help. These satellite tents are used for initial evaluation and treatment of patients but are too small to keep patients who need to be observed for an extended period of time. When a patient is combative, and in need of additional care, we'll be called to transport them to our primary medical tent. That tent is larger with more staff, sometimes including doctors. The smaller tents are staffed with only one or two people so a combative patient can cause quite a bit of chaos and can possibly endanger staff and others around them. That was our concern based on what we had heard over the radio.

When we arrived, we saw a petite young woman of perhaps 17 or 18 sitting in the stair chair that had been used to bring her from the stage to the tent. She was strapped securely to the chair, as is common with all patients to be sure they are safe for transport. An EMT stood on either side of her. She was calm and well-behaved.

"Is this our patient?" I asked.

"Yep, that's her."

"You called us for her?" I wasn't sure this was the same person we had heard over the radio.

"Yeah, she is a pain in the ass."

Looking at her sitting there, it didn't make sense to us that she needed to go to the main tent, but it didn't take long for the reason to become clear.

When we released the chair straps, she jumped up, yelled "I've got to go," and attempted to run off. We grabbed her, got her into the front seat of our medical cart, and put a seat belt around her. I was driving, so my partner slid her to the middle and sat next to her so she couldn't jump out.

Unfortunately, either the bumps along the dirt path or the vibrations of the motor underneath her provided too much stimulation and she began to writhe around in erotic pleasure. It was all we could do to keep her in the seat, off the floor, and in the cart.

She also began to repeatedly shriek, "Give it to me, give it to me, give it to me!" I managed to alert the main tent supervisor that we were coming in with a patient who needed to go straight into the ambulance to the hospital. When they questioned me, I simply keyed the mic open as she screamed and moaned. That got their attention.

As we pulled up to the tent, others were in the process of getting a stretcher from the ambulance. Our patient had managed to squirm her way down the seat and had her feet on the dashboard. When we came to a stop, she arched her back and threw her legs out in front of her, hitting the windshield with enough force to pop it out of its holding clips. One of our paramedics managed to catch it to keep it from breaking. At that point, the easiest way to get her on the stretcher was to simply pass her lying down through the open windshield onto the stretcher.

I learned later that her orgasmic adventure had continued the entire trip to the ER, although this time in four-point restraints.

Nurse Flasher

I was a new EMT working a three-day heavy metal event that took place outside within a sports stadium. I was new to the company providing the medical staff and had not met many of my colleagues. My partner and I were inside the stadium when we got a call for an intoxicated person on the stadium concourse.

We found a young woman sitting against the wall who did indeed appear to be very intoxicated. She was alert but not even close to being oriented. Her vital signs were normal, but her speech was slurred. It took some effort, but she was finally able to tell us that, in fact, she was "fucked up" and that her friends had left her. She then leaned over and vomited on my shoes. Well, nice to meet you too.

Security helped us get her onto our stair chair and we took her to the first aid room manned by Joe, a relatively new paramedic. I had not worked with him before, but he seemed pretty competent. What did I know? I was new and naïve.

Joe did a full assessment on her while I tried to contact her fiancé to ask him to come pick her up. As she lay on the exam bed, she told us she was a nurse in an ER at a hospital in the area. She was very "friendly" and, having vomited, now felt quite frisky.

"Do you need me to take off my shirt?" she asked.

"No ma'am, you can keep your shirt on," I said.

"Are you sure? I can take off my shirt." She started to unbutton it.

"No ma'am, please keep your shirt on."

"But you need to see my boobs."

This continued for some time with us repeatedly telling her we did *not* need to see her breasts and that we did *not* want her to take her shirt off. Finally, Joe had enough.

"Look, I play on the other team," he said, "so I have no interest in your boobs."

As Joe shared with the patient his *position*, I explained to her fiancé via phone that he needed to come pick her up or we would transfer her to the hospital. It was all I could do to maintain any level of professionalism with him as I listened to Joe's conversation. To his credit, it all ended well. The shirt stayed on, the fiancé arrived to take her home, and Joe and I became good friends and colleagues.

Once paramedics assess for any life-threatening conditions, they move on to a more detailed secondary assessment. We use a systematic process to get important information about the patient: symptoms, allergies, medications, past medical history, last oral intake, events leading to current problem, and the following about their issue:

Onset

Provocation

Quality of pain

Region/radiation of pain

Severity

Time or how long they have had their symptoms.

This is one of the earliest skills I learned as an EMT. Unless there is a specific reason, disrobing is never required.

Room Service
As Told by John (Paramedic)

I was a 54-year-old veteran of countless musical festivals, sporting events, and other large gatherings over my 30-plus years as a paramedic. I thought I had seen it all, done it all, and gotten the T-shirt. But even I was surprised by what happened to me at a particular weekend event.

We were working at a two-day outdoor music festival in August. It was a pretty typical event, featuring mostly hard-rock musicians and a local crowd. I came across a woman who had been brought into our busy medical tent because of a fall, but she appeared to have only scrapes and bruises. The tent was busy at that moment so I jumped in, as we all would, and helped to take care of her. She was in her 30s, attractive with long dark hair, and very friendly. That was not unusual at these events.

As we talked while I cleaned her wounds, she told me that she was from Oklahoma and was staying at a nearby hotel. I didn't think there were many people like her in attendance, but it wasn't a total surprise that she was visiting. As I cleaned and bandaged her cuts and scrapes, we had a normal conversation. For a while.

"My hotel is just down the street here. Very close," she said.

"Well, that's convenient." I hadn't picked up on things yet.

"Yep, I'm in room 301, in case you want to stop by."

"Uhhh…" I was a bit speechless at this. I was married, working, and she was my patient. It would have been inappropriate on many levels to accept her offer. In addition, while I like to think I am a quite handsome firefighter paramedic, the truth is I am no Tom Cruise. And I was close to twice her age. In addition, she was, in all likelihood, not sober.

I smiled and thanked her but declined to join her in her hotel room. She shrugged and left the medical tent to return to the music. As fate would have it, I ran into her several more times that evening, and each time she reminded me of where she was staying. Her interest went from awkward to humorous with each passing request. I did see her again the next day, but fortunately she had either sobered up or lost interest. I did not get another invitation.

Happy Butterfly

You often hear emergency room nurses speak of "frequent flyers," patients whom they see in the ER on a regular basis. Some of them have legitimate medical issues that cause repeat visits; for others, it can sometimes seem like a game.

I had never seen a frequent flyer at a weekend festival until I met this young lady. At least once every day of the festival, she made her way into the medical tent for some reason. On the last night of the event, I responded to a call of a woman hanging from a tree. When I arrived, I recognized her immediately.

Hanging not from her hands, but by her arms, this frequent flyer swung back and forth, declaring, "I'm a social butterfly and I'm swinging from tree to tree."

I was not really in the mood for her antics at this point and told her to get in the cart.

When we arrived at the medical tent, we walked in and saw a young man already on a cot screaming that he was having a "penile seizure." To address this seizure, he began to overtly masturbate in the medical tent.

Yes, you read that correctly.

Obviously, we put a stop to it, but our female social butterfly felt badly for this young man. She sat down next to him and began to stroke his face and hair. A nurse noticed and came over to check on Madam Butterfly, which was all I needed to get out of that mess.

A short time later, I was back in the tent with another patient and noticed that the young man with the penile seizure and the social butterfly were now both crying. I don't know why they were crying, and honestly, I didn't really care at that point. But as luck would have it, the young man had a cure for the tears. He took out his phone and began playing the Pharrell Williams song *Happy*.

"Because I'm happyyyy. Clap along if you feel like happiness is the truth."

With that, they were both all smiles.

There is a cultural tradition at some music festivals to give people you meet "kandi." This is usually a simple bracelet made of beads or stones, often homemade, that participants wear on their arms. They are exchanged as a sign of thanks, gratitude, or affection.

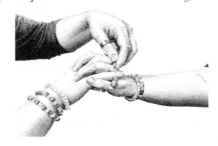

I have had several people give me kandi as thanks for my service to them, and it's the only appropriate sign of affection to accept from a patient.

Fun Run
As Told by Jerone (Paramedic)

Bath salts, not the kind we put in bathtubs, were a serious problem. Sold as a powder or crystals, these "salts," also known as the zombie drug, are swallowed, snorted, or injected. They are made of a material called cathinone, which is similar to meth and Molly. It increases feelings of happiness, a desire for social interaction, and a person's sex drive. The drug can also cause hostility and hallucinations, as I found out.

Not far from our medical tent was a driveway and a parking lot. Security called to let us know there was a woman running up and down the drive screaming. Because of her crazed behavior, they wanted us to evaluate her before they did anything. When I arrived, I saw a rather obese young woman running from one end of the drive to the other. Most notable was that she was doing it with one hand down her shorts, screaming about the pleasure she was giving herself. She was quite vocal and very descriptive about what she was doing and how much she was enjoying herself. I looked at the security guys; they shrugged.

We tried to calm her down, but she was in a groove and running like the energizer bunny. As we tried to talk to her, she finally stopped and lay down under a tree where she went into full-on public masturbation. I really didn't want to interfere and get her running again, and she *did* seem to be enjoying herself, so we let her finish what she was doing and then sedated her for a much-needed trip to the ER.

At about the same time, we got another call from security alerting us to a guy running around smashing into people. My partner and I responded and found a large, well-built guy running and bowling over anyone he could. He was absolutely body slamming people. It turns out he was the partner of the masturbator. Apparently, they had enjoyed some bath salts together and had had very dramatic, yet totally different reactions to the drug. It took several of us, but we were able to restrain and sedate him so he could join his girlfriend for a date in the ER.

Let's Trade
As Told by Jon (EMT)

On one beautiful day, I found myself at the front of a stage which was sandwiched between the city skyline and a pristine lake. My job was watching for anyone who needed help, or for security to call me to assist with someone. A young woman at the front of the crowd along the fence caught my attention.

"Hey, nice shirt," she told me.

"Thank you."

"Can I get one?"

It was a simple T-shirt with the name of our company that identified me as part of the medical team. It also gave me authority to enter areas off limits to the general public. There was no way I could give her, or anyone, the shirt.

"No, sorry. It's my work shirt," I said. "I can't give them away."

Still she persisted, telling me that she really liked it and would be very happy if I gave one to her. She was very friendly and not being obnoxious about it, but I had to politely explain that I could not give her a shirt. She then went way past friendly and indicated just *how* much she wanted a shirt.

"Come on. You give me a shirt and I'll give you the best blowjob you've ever had."

Wow. I mean, *wow*. I was at least her father's age and had never been confused for a male model. I admit, there was a small part of me that was flattered, for about a second. I knew, of course, that this was all drug or alcohol-induced "friendliness." It was also pretty awkward since my young EMT partner was right beside me.

It goes without saying that it would have been extremely inappropriate for me to accept her offer. I politely declined and moved to the other side of the stage.

THE PATIENT IS WHERE?

"I smell the smelly smell of something that smells smelly." – SpongeBob

One of the absolute necessities at music festivals, and other outdoor events, is the porta-potty. You see them in rows lining the fences with long lines of angry users complaining that there are never

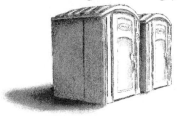

enough. By the second or third day of an event, some of these plastic waste collection points are well-used and less than pleasing. And of course, when someone isn't feeling well, they often go to the closest bathroom, in this case the porta-potty.

For anyone who has ever worked at an outdoor event, you know the absolute worst call to get is a potty call. "Team 3, go to stage one for a sick person in the porta-potties." *Nooooo!* So distasteful are these calls that gamesmanship can often occur to get out of responding.

In one case, my partner and I were in our cart parked next to another team when the call came in.

"Team 3, respond to the porta-potty by campground two for a sick person."

Well, I was Team 3 and as I groaned and shook my head at our bad luck, the other team – Team 5 – howled with laughter.

My partner, a seasoned veteran of these festivals, didn't flinch. "Team 5 says they will take that. They are en route," he told dispatch.

I nearly fell out of our cart laughing as Team 5 drove off to the call, swearing loudly at my smiling partner. When we caught up with them later, they were busy hosing down their cart.

Slip Sliding

I was working with a younger yet more experienced partner when a young woman came to us and told us her sick friend was in the porta-potty across the street from us. Hoping she was just resting, or maybe vomiting, we went to check on her. What we found was easily the worst, most disgusting call of my career.

Oh, and that newfound compassion and understanding I've been talking about? Not this time.

The friend was in a large handicap-accessible potty, which was big enough to lie down in – which she was. She appeared to be in her early 20s, wearing shorts and a tank top. Lying primarily on her back, she was breathing, but was otherwise completely unresponsive. This was day three of the festival and it was hot, so the floor was not fresh and clean. In fact, it was wet, muddy, and smeared with urine, vomit, and who knows what else. Some of it belonged to our patient, and some of it didn't. And there she was, passed out in the middle of it.

In my time working in healthcare, there have only been two times when I gagged and almost vomited. The first was in an emergency room when a patient whose system was backed up from a blocked colon vomited into the basin I was holding. It was so vile that I gagged, turned my head away, and had to breathe through my mouth to make it through that moment. This potty call was the second time.

As I walked in and saw the patient, I immediately turned and walked out. The smell was indescribable. I prayed I would not puke in front of the crowd that had gathered. It would not be a good look for the medical staff to be seen losing breakfast. My partner began to swear and we both just looked at each other. We knew we had to attend to this woman, assess her, and transport her to a medical tent. We had gloves, but no masks to hide the smell. It was enough to make me question my career choice.

We recruited two security guards to help us get her onto our backboard so we could put her on our cart. But as we grabbed her arms and legs to lift her, our hands slipped off her skin. We could not get any kind of grip on her thanks to all the sloppy mess that clung to her flesh. We made several attempts but no luck. She was just too slippery to grasp. She also was big enough that we could not lift her by her trunk, so we were at a loss until my wise partner came up with a solution.

He went across the street to our medical tent and borrowed a blanket. We put the blanket on the floor and slid it underneath her. We then picked her up by the blanket and moved her to our cart and then to the medical tent where the doctors were not thrilled to see us.

The young woman who had alerted us to this situation was in shock at her friend's condition.

"How much did she have to drink?" I asked her.

"She only had two vodkas," the friend replied.

Right, it's always *just two*.

It was 11:15 a.m. The music had not yet started.

Her expensive festival tickets were as wasted as she was.

Splish Splash
As Told by Ryan (EMT)

One of the issues I see often at music festivals is young adults being careless with their valuables. The two most common items I see lost or stolen are cell phones and sunglasses. In most cases, by the time you realize you have lost the item, it's too late to find it. But in one special situation, my intoxicated patient gave it his best shot, with surprising results.

My partner and I were called to the porta-potties at an outdoor three-day festival. When we arrived, we could hear what sounded like splashing water. We knocked and called for the person inside, but he did not answer us or make any attempt to open the door. But we continued to hear sloshing and it was clear that this person was the source.

I had learned how to take a door off a porta-potty in case of an emergency; it's surprisingly easy. When we didn't get a response from the occupant, and it was clear that all or part of him was in some type of fluid, I removed the door to see what was going on. Inside was a young man who had inserted himself into the hole of the toilet face-first, with one arm digging and splashing around in the muck. And whatever you are thinking as you read this, we thought the same thing when we saw it.

"Hey buddy, what are you doing?" I asked.

"What?"

"What are you doing down there?"

We grabbed him and pulled him out of the mess to talk to him.

"I think I lost my sunglasses down there," he said. "They're really expensive."

I had something to tell him. "Dude, your sunglasses are clipped to your shirt."

"Oh. Damn." He grinned like we had just made his day.

Because he was obviously in an altered mental state and had been playing in poop, we wanted to take him to the medical tent to be evaluated. But under the circumstances, we really didn't want to put him on our stair chair. Fortunately, he was able to walk with us the short distance there. He told us his name was Danny.

One of the medics who was in the tent said to the young man, "Boy, Danny, you're having a shitty day." Medical humor.

Danny just nodded and was taken to sleep it off.

We didn't stick around, but at the end of the night when we went back to the medical tent, I saw Danny's sunglasses on the table. Danny was long gone. I couldn't help but laugh at the irony. Danny, in his intoxicated state, had dug through a nasty porta-potty looking for sunglasses that he hadn't lost and then lost those very sunglasses when he left the medical tent. Precious.

Because the sunglasses were going to be thrown away, I took them as a reminder of my now infamous patient. I would like to say I hoped to run into Danny and return them, but the odds of that were low, and they were nice glasses.

About four months later, I went to an outdoor food stand to order some lunch. The guy who served me my sandwich looked at me and said, "You look really familiar."

Well, I'm a white, Irish guy so half the world looks like me.

"No, I know you. Where did you get those sunglasses?" the server said.

I gave him an abbreviated version of how I came to be wearing the glasses.

He looked at me and said, "I'm Danny."

I mean, what are the chances, right? In a city of three million people, I buy lunch from a patient who had been digging around in sewage.

I gave Danny his sunglasses back and then threw out all of my food. I mean, I knew where his hands had been.

When a patient is acting crazy or has an altered mental status, it may be because they are drunk or on drugs. But they may also have hypoglycemia, or low blood sugar, which can be a deadly condition. The symptoms can look very similar to an intoxicated person. As a result, we always check the person's glucose level. Even when I'm sure the person is drunk or high, I still check. It's easy and inexpensive and can be lifesaving.

Squatty Potty
As Told by Jake (Paramedic)

I was working at a very large festival and was assigned with another EMT to a field team, meaning we were out in the crowd with a supply bag and a stair chair ready to respond to calls in our area. A couple of people came across the street towards us.

"You guys are medical, right?"

"Yep, what's going on?"

"Our friend has been in the porta-potty for a long time and she isn't answering us."

"Was she sick?"

"No, she just went to pee."

We were close, so we followed them to the row of portable johns and found the one she had entered. She didn't respond to our knocking or our calls, so we were concerned for her wellbeing. A nearby police officer helped us get the door open and when I looked inside, I was stunned. There was the young woman *in the potty*. And by in the potty, I mean her head, arms, and one leg were sticking up through the seat, with the rest of her below the seat. I really didn't know what to say to her.

Other than being very embarrassed and uncomfortable, she was fine. We were able to help her up and out of the very non-sanitary sanitary waste. It turns out, she went to use the bathroom but did not want to sit on the seat, so she had attempted to stand above it and squat, allowing her to go without actually touching anything with her bottom.

As luck would have it though, one of her feet had slipped and down she had gone, with one leg through the opening and the other caught above her head outside the opening. The music was loud enough that no one could hear her calls for help. I can't imagine those few moments for her.

She ended up being fine and with quite a story to tell. The only lingering effects were the smell she carried and the blue dye from the potty that covered one of her legs.

Just Chilln'
As Told by Nathan (EMT)

My team was called to a porta-potty by the company that was hired to clean them. They had a row roped off and were moving down the line sucking the contents into their truck. But one of the units was still occupied and the person in it would not come out. We knocked without response, so we eventually took the door off and found a teenager curled in a ball on the seat, completely naked. Not only was he not wearing any clothes, but there were no clothes with him. It was just him, curled up, and naked.

"Hey, what's going on?" I asked.

"Just chillin'," he said sheepishly

"Okay, but you can't chill in there," I replied.

"Well, do you have any pants I can wear?"

I felt bad for this poor kid, but we do not carry extra clothes with us. Instead, we cut leg holes in a big black plastic bag, which gave him at least a small amount of decency while he went on his way. We never found out why he was naked nor did we ever locate his clothes. Mystery unsolved.

WHAT HAVE I LEARNED?

"It's fine to celebrate success, but it is more important to heed the lessons of failure." – Bill Gates

By now, you have some sense of the experiences that transformed me from a white-collar lawyer and business executive to a dirt-under-my-nails, hands-on paramedic. But that story is incomplete without discussing the mistakes I've made.

Throughout my career, some of the most important things I've learned have come from making mistakes. If you can admit your mistake and understand why you made it, you can then learn how to correct it and prevent it from happening again. In business, mistakes might cost money or anger a customer. Unfortunately, for an EMT or paramedic, making mistakes can have more tragic consequences. Therefore, it is essential that we learn from them.

I was working as a paramedic at a local distance race and was deployed on one of the teams on the course. My partner and I were assigned a spot not far from the finish. It was a beautiful morning for everything except running a distance race. In fact, it was one of the first warm days of the year, which meant the runners had not had a chance to acclimate to the heat after a cold winter. The course ran through a beautiful park filled with trees but also had numerous areas unprotected from the sun. Unsurprisingly, a number of the participants met trouble.

For most of the race, the runners ran along a bike/walking path. The return portion of the course gave way to a beautiful view of a lake but was also the most exposed, offering little protection from the sun.

We had just returned from a call for a man who had suffered a seizure. When we had found him, he had been sitting along the path in a post-seizure state, confused and unable to process what was happening. As we had placed him onto a stretcher, he had become slightly more aware and coherent. We had transferred him to the ambulance to be taken to the ER.

When we returned to our designated spot, a young woman stopped in front of us, staggered for a few steps, and then nearly fell into the grass. Because she was only a few yards from us, we were with her almost immediately. I estimated her age to be in the late 20s; she appeared to be very fit. She was able to tell me her name, but when I asked if she knew where she was, she was unable to answer, despite looking directly at an obvious landmark. This should have been my clue, but I missed it.

As I assessed her, I found her skin hot to the touch and she was sweating. These were both possibly significant findings, but in this case, neither were unexpected after running for more than an hour. I don't remember what her blood pressure was, but it didn't mean much to me at the time. I recall her heartrate was fast, but again, she had been running. So, while I knew I needed to get her to the medical tent, I didn't recognize the biggest sign of danger: her confusion.

All of this took place in a matter of a minute or two, and there was a lot of activity around us. The band continued to play while fans cheered the runners who ran by just feet from us. It was a scene of a lot of activity. Another runner, a man in his 50s, stopped, wobbled, and sat down just a few feet from us. He had that glassy-eyed appearance of someone who was unsure of who and where he was. So now, in the space of about 10 feet on either side of a running path filled with runners and lined by spectators, I had two patients who needed my attention.

At that point, I had completed my paramedic training but was not yet licensed to practice as a medic. I really wasn't authorized to have started an IV on either of them in the field if I had thought of it. But I certainly knew how. I wish I could say that is why I didn't, but the truth was, with everything happening around me, I never thought of it. I knew they were suffering from heat illness but failed to understand just how serious it was, particularly for the female patient. I learned later that if a patient is confused or altered at all, assume it is heat stroke, the most serious and deadly type of heat illness, and treat it with appropriate urgency.

Instead, after making sure they were able to swallow safely, we gave both of them a bottle of cold water, helped them to our golf cart, and set off for the medical area. The man sat next to me as I drove; the woman sat on the back seat with my partner. It was only then that I realized I didn't know where I was going. In my haste to get out to our positions that morning, I had been too casual and thus was unprepared. At this point, it was my heart rate that was fast, and it's likely I was now sweating as well.

Even after I radioed for the location, I didn't know how to get there. It wasn't complicated or far; I simply hadn't taken the time to learn the best route and how to navigate some gates and security closures. There I was, with two sick patients in my care and I was fumbling to get them where they needed to be. If you are a parent and have ever felt badly because you did not know what to do to help your sick child, you can understand my emotions at the time.

I finally sorted out my directions and we headed quickly to the spot, but even then, things did not go smoothly. To add to my concern, the patient next to me leaned away from the cart and began vomiting, profusely. As I drove, I held onto him, trying to keep him from falling out. My partner in the back seat was doing her best to keep the other patient stable, reminding me that she was pretty sick.

This could not end soon enough for me.

I was responsible for the lives of these two people who had come out to have fun and run a race, and I was making a mess of it. The result of all of this was that we took several minutes longer than necessary getting our patients to the higher level of care they needed. I felt sick, embarrassed, worried for my patients, and generally incompetent.

Fortunately, this story ends well. I saw the woman later when I transported her to a waiting ambulance. She had received IV fluid and been cooled with ice packs. She looked much better and was more alert and oriented. She went to the

ER for further evaluation and treatment and made a total recovery.

I was told the man was given cold water and some wet sponges to cool himself and after being evaluated, had been released to his wife in good condition.

As for me, I learned several valuable lessons about being prepared to do my job and staying calm and focused on the patient in front of me.

It was a wake-up call – what I do can be fun until it's not.

TELL ME AGAIN, WHY DO I DO THIS?

"Oh…there won't be any money, but when you die on your deathbed, you will receive total consciousness. So I got that goin' for me. Which is nice." – Bill Murray, Caddyshack

At this point, at least some of you must be wondering just why the heck I do this. It's okay, I get it. Even my family thinks I am either crazy or suffering a mid-life (late-life?) crisis. I am forbidden from sharing these kinds of stories with them. My wife also worries at times about my safety, even though she knows I am very cautious.

For many in this field, the emotional strain caused by what we witness is debilitating. But for me, and I'm sure most of my colleagues, the best answer to "why" has to do with the rewards of a job well-done. I'm not talking about financial rewards since many EMTs and paramedics are paid only slightly more than minimum wage, but the personal rewards. It sounds trite, I know. But there is an immense sense of self-satisfaction when your actions help another person most in need.

I share this final short story from my friend and colleague John, a paramedic, because it illustrates why we put up with the loud music, the vomit, the crazy antics, and the long days or nights.

As Told by John (Paramedic)

Most people in the EMS community would not consider this much of a story. But to me, it was one of the most meaningful moments in my long career as an EMT and paramedic.

We were working at a large event when a mom brought her young boy into our medical tent. He was perhaps five or six-years-old and had fallen off a golf cart that he had either been riding in or playing on. When I looked at his arm, I saw an obvious deformity which suggested it was broken. Officially, only an x-ray can tell if a bone is truly broken, but I was pretty sure this little man's imaging would show a fracture.

I don't recall if he was crying at the time, but he was

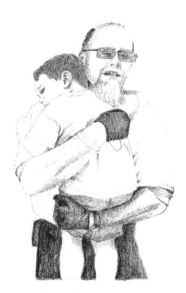

obviously scared and in some amount of distress. As was my habit, I got on my knees to be at his level and told him that I was going to help his arm feel better and then give him a ride in our very cool ambulance. He seemed all right with that. I splinted his arm the best I could and wrapped it to keep it secure, all the while talking to him to keep his mind off his injury.

As his mom led him away toward the ambulance, he stopped, ran back to me, and gave me a big hug. For an old, weary paramedic who had seen too much tragedy, it was one of my best "saves" ever.

LOOKING BACK

"The only reason you should ever look back is to see how far you've come."
– Unknown

I've been working at music festivals for more than three years. I look forward to them each summer and will continue to work at them for as long as I am able. As I reflect on my experiences, I realize how much they have changed me. I knew little about music festivals or the party-drug culture and I would have frowned on my daughters participating in it. The "corporate" me would have never approved.

But I have watched tens of thousands of young adults at these festivals partying responsibly and having the time of their lives. I have seen young men and women of all backgrounds dancing together and cheering, unbound by the inhibitions I grew up with. It intrigues me. Clearly, there is something to these events that makes them so popular. I still do not advocate illegal drug use, but I have grown to better understand why some people do; I wish only for them to use wisely and safely.

I have also become more tolerant of others and how their decisions impact me. I've been spit on, coughed on, thrown up on, and had to clean just about every bodily fluid imaginable from my patients and myself. I can't say that I like it, but it's just a part of the job. And it pales in comparison to the satisfaction I get from being able to comfort a patient or relieve their pain.

I have ridden in ambulances with sick children, patients having heart attacks, and victims of car accidents. I've performed CPR on a kitchen floor and in the ER as a patient's spouse watched and cried. I've given medication to relieve pain, reduce anxiety, and correct a dangerous heart condition. I've held the hands of a frightened elderly patient as we took her to the hospital and I've helped those who have fallen and could not get up. In each case, the satisfaction of providing care for the patient is what drove me to the next call.

At music festivals, that sense of satisfaction is combined with the very real energy and joy reverberating through festival goers and I feel like I am right where I am supposed to be. I am blessed to have had a great professional career that allows me now to do what I do. I'm not changing the world, but I'm making it a little better for my patients in that moment. I like that.

Perhaps the biggest difference is how my family sees me. I was the serious dad and husband, the one who felt responsible for climbing the corporate ladder and providing for my family. I probably wasn't always that much fun. My wife and daughters now sometimes wonder what happened to that conservative, no-nonsense lawyer; I'm sure, even now, their bewilderment is still present.

Where did this tolerant, fun-loving guy come from?

I just tell them… Molly did it.

If you wish to donate to **The First Responders Children's Foundation**, please visit their website at:
www. https://1strcf.org/

ACKNOWLEDGMENTS

When I decided to write this book, I had no idea how much was involved or how many people I would need to support me. I do now. My deepest thanks start with my wife Sandy and my daughters Jenn and Mara who have endured endless stories of my adventures and my obsession with the details of this book. I could not have written this book without their help and support. They have made this a better book and me a better person.

My editor Kara Scrivener at Emerging Ink Solutions was the calm voice in my ear when I was anxious and uncertain. She made this book and the process of writing it so much better. If you are thinking of writing a book, talk to Kara.

My friend Melanie Goldish who I met sitting on a plane read and reviewed some of my earliest versions and never failed to give me both honest feedback and needed encouragement.

So many of my friends and colleagues contributed to this book, either through their stories or helping me verify details and get the medicine right. Thank you to Jerone Lucas, Pam Szott, Josh Armstrong, Jake Thornton, Lindsay Olszewski, John Schmidt, Colleen Clark, Nathan Poling, Jon Bjork, Ryan Ward, Sarah Goldstein, and others who wish to remain anonymous. You all know better than most the joy and sadness of our profession. Your contributions gave this book depth that it would otherwise not have had.

Lacy Colligan was my first contact for advice after she wrote and published her book and she shared many very valuable resources with me. To the countless others who shared my excitement, tolerated my incessant chatter, and graciously turned their heads before rolling their eyes during this process – you helped in ways I'll never be able to express.

Jennifer Andos at Paperfish Creative gave generously of her time and talent, helping me with my social media and communications. Her commitment to first responders is genuine and I was honored to have her assistance.

I benefitted from some truly amazing educators in the process of becoming a paramedic. Chris Dunn, Mike Gentile, Jen Dyer and Kourtney Chesney not only taught me the skills I needed, but modeled the way a high-quality medical professional cares for patients. My training was re-enforced outside the classroom by my preceptors on the ambulance Rich Spellman and Frank Doll. I am grateful for their invaluable assistance.

And Matt Schipper, it all started with you. You gave me a chance and I am forever thankful for that.

ABOUT THE AUTHOR

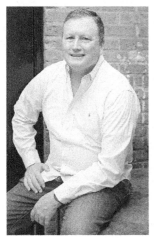

Jim is a paramedic in the Chicagoland area after a career-change from a lawyer and business executive. He has a degree in Criminology from Indiana University of Pennsylvania and a law degree from The Pennsylvania State University, Dickinson School of Law.

He and his wife Sandy have two grown daughters, Jenn and Mara. Jim spends his spare time reading, watching movies with his wife, and cheering on his Pittsburgh Steelers. This is his first book.

Made in the USA
Monee, IL
27 January 2021

58261448R00059